THE WRONG PRESCRIPTION

ABOUT THE AUTHOR

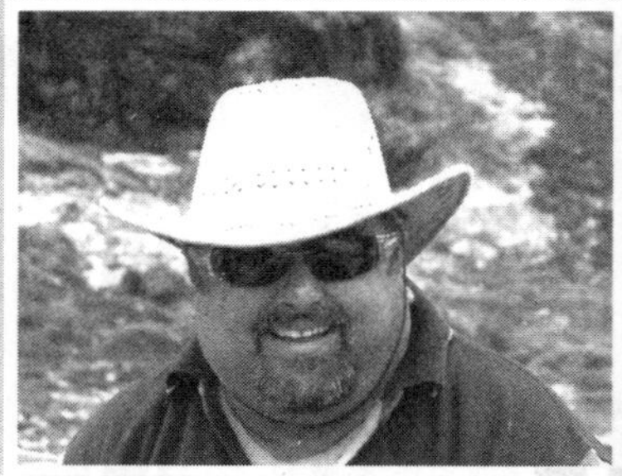

Imagine Samuel Pickwick with a scalpel and you have Dr Manoj Kapoor. The amiable doctor, in today's world, is the very antithesis of what is generally thought about his tribe. It is assumed that the doctors are a gruff, business-like lot. But he is a boy scout among his fraternity with a broad, infectious smile playing about his lips.

His formative years were spent in various cities and countries. Initial schooling started from St Columbus School in Delhi and then he studied in a school in Kabul. The son of an IFS officer and a teacher mother, he cleared his middle school from Delhi Public school, R.K. Puram. High school was completed in the state of Virginia in U.S.A. From then on M.P. Shah medical college, Jamnagar became the alma mater. Intermittent tenures of work and training took him to Delhi but since the last 20 years he has been in Ahmedabad.

Being fond of a lot of other activities besides promoting his profession Manoj dedicated his non working hours to serving the NGO'S. As a matter of fact, he held many posts in different non government organizations and served as Area Chairman, Area-3, Round Table India. The thrust of this NGO was on primary education. He also worked with Pratham and Blind People's Association and the Rotary movement. Diligent and sincere work in these organizations helped him mature and learn a lot about life. His global upbringing had already taught him to observe life at close quarters and the gentleman's efforts did not go in vain.

Manoj has a facile pen and a matching warm heart. A keen observer of men and matters, the doctor cocks a snoot at his errant compeers in an inoffensive way. As he himself says in his narrative, his intention is not to condemn them but to remind them of their duties.

His wife Parul , a leading Gynaecologist, completed her master's from M.P.Shah medical college, Jamnagar. After 2 years of rural service, the couple started a hospital in Ahmedabad in 1991, on what till the other day used to be outskirts of the city of Ahmedabad. They aptly named it 'Samarpan' – services dedicated to the suffering humanity.

Many are the qualities of the head and the heart that endear him to his numerous patients. One of them, Varanasi Rama Murthy, a senior journalist, has hit the nail on the head when he says, "It is extremely difficult not to like Dr Manoj Kapoor."

THE WRONG PRESCRIPTION

A SAGA OF THE MEDICAL PROFESSION AND ITS PASSAGE THROUGH TIME

Dr. Manoj Kapoor, M.S

GOOD TIMES

GOOD TIMES BOOKS PVT. LTD.
New Delhi (India)
www.goodtimesbooks.com

Published by
GOOD TIMES BOOKS PVT. LTD.
H-13, Bali Nagar, New Delhi-110 015 (INDIA)
Phones: +91-11-25913301, 45069086 Fax: +91-11-45069086
Email : info@goodtimesbooks.com
Website : www.goodtimesbooks.com

First Good Times Edition 2011
ISBN-13 : 978-93-806192-5-5

Typeset in 13 pts. Venetian 301 BT
by Good Times Design Cell

Printed in India at
Salasar Imaging Systems

This book is dedicated to my wife Parul, my sons Anshuman and Rohan, and my teachers who taught me surgery and the nobility of the profession.

I am indebted to the patients who had faith in me and all those who supported me in my life!

CONTENTS

ACKNOWLEDGMENTS

A thank you speech or an acknowledgment is one of the most difficult things to write. Life is a learning curve. Everything and everybody around me has taught me something. The possibility that one might end up highlighting the contribution of a few and excluding others makes this exercise difficult.

Keeping this in mind I want to be very careful not to tread on anyone's sentiments. I start off by thanking all the friends and acquaintances who believe in me and have consistently boosted my morale and propped me up whenever I have been low. They may not be directly associated with my writing this book, but I am proud to admit that their faith has kept me going. At times, my tone and language may have hurt many a person along the way, but the ones who have stayed with me are the ones who have understood me. I have no qualms about admitting that I have better bonding with ladies, who have been my pillars of strength and who have had more faith in me and my capabilities than my male friends. These ladies are my mother and my wife, my kid sister and the lady friends in the medical college, followed by a few friends' wives. I hold them all in high esteem and thank them from the bottom of my heart.

The one person I am deeply indebted to is Mr. Varanasi Ramamurthy, who edited this book. A retired senior editor of the

Times of India, he still leads an active life and has kept in touch with his profession remarkably well. Sharvari, a close friend's daughter who recently graduated from 'Shristi' did the sketches with my younger son, Rohan, who joined Symbiosis, Pune in July of 2010 for his Bachelor's in Media and Communication. Two ladies put their heart and soul into giving this book the final finesse. Smita Premchander and Dolly Saxena spared valuable time from their busy schedules to guide me and give this book the class that a good book aspires to. Both these ladies have their own busy vocations to attend to. A select few friends read the manuscript and gave me inputs which were very valuable. Prarit, Saroj Mullick and Dr Behuria are friends who helped me in finding a pan India publisher and taking care of many other formalities. Dr Parthasarathy, Director at CEPT, and a friend to me, finally introduced me to Mr. Devashish Mittal, Publisher at Good Times Books Pvt. Ltd. I am highly indebted to both these gentlemen to have done their best for me, and that too beyond the call of duty. The whole publication team of Good Times has done a phenomenal job in weaving this book into its present form.

Parul, my wife of 21 years and a friend of 30 years is my driving force. She has encouraged me silently and steadily towards higher goals in life, and is my better half in the truest sense of the word. While she hates my tongue when I am angry, she loves me for my vulnerability I think, and she has been the pillar, the foundation and everything for me. Anshuman and Rohan are my two sons, who have grown up into my best friends and have been with me through thick and thin.

Om Gam Ganapataye Namah

LAUGHTER IS THE BEST MEDICINE

Doctors are not supposed to be physically overpowering personalities. A six-pack doctor is a rarity, though not an impossibility. How do they fight their battles or settle their grievances? Certainly not by giving wrong prescriptions! The calling they have chosen for their livelihood teaches them the virtues of compassion, restraint, patience and forbearance, facilitated by knowledge and continuous learning. And these very virtues help them overcome their setbacks. Or do they? After all we are only human. A book of this kind is one way of addressing this issue. Working at times with sad and demanding situations takes its toll on doctors. If humour and wit get deficient in the medical world, it starts to show on the mental health of the doctor. The life of a doctor is sweet and sour. A few episodes suffice to show this. The sweetness in life is when everything is going as per the perfect plan and sourness is when nothing happens as per plan.

A doctor friend of mine was aware of his senior's competence, or rather lack of it, in certain areas of surgical art. As chance would have it, during a two-month vacation period in their medical college, this very professor took over as the temporary head of the unit. A patient who was suffering from multiple diseases, all of them very critical in nature, was awaiting surgery. The professor who took charge of the unit got excited and asked the junior doctors to post this complicated patient for surgery. No amount of excuses to postpone given by the junior doctors could change his mind. Fearing the worst, my friend went to the extent of counseling the patient that he was in a precarious condition and that these kinds of surgeries are better left to the specialists. But the patient had probably got tired of waiting for his turn to get operated and refused to heed the advice. Aware of the ultimate fate which the patient was unknowingly facing, a concerned doctor, daringly witty to say the least, gave the pre-operative prescription to the patient's relative. Along with the genuine list of surgical consumables, a list of things required for cremation under the Hindu religion was added. The patient's relative responded with a startled expression asking for an explanation for the 'wrong prescription'. Our friend coolly explained that "these things will be required after the surgery. Any unpreparedness at the time of mourning leads to chaos and it is better to be prepared." While we, the group of junior doctors, were laughing and smirking, the patient's relative got livid. He was upset but also intelligent enough to get the message. He took the patient away immediately. Next morning the senior doctor was told that the patient had absconded. The patient lived and came back later to get operated on by a more competent person and thus survived. Whether or not it was a wrong prescription is an answer which only the patient can give.

This book is about where and why we doctors went wrong and are going wrong and whether it is entirely our mistake or an ill of the system that is evolving. The more serious matters shall be taken up in the various chapters of this book. Real life incidents, funny incidents and anecdotes lessen the misery around the doctors. The hospital and the suffering patients can take a toll on anybody's mental health, but these funny incidents enliven the proceedings.

The medical profession spawns many adult jokes, some of them nauseating. Under the grim-faced, serious-looking and often bespectacled doctor lies the farceur – alternately subtle and crude, at times very abstruse too. The SOS for the healer, in and around the world of suffering, is this farcical side. No! The wit is not on the hapless patients. The jest is on self, peers and seniors. Performance in adversity starts from the student days. Survival of the fittest is the order of the day in the profession of healing. Mental fitness and wit are mutually non-reciprocal. Humour in any form takes shape then. Respected professors are instrumental in providing fodder to the gossip.

I vividly remember the time when as freshers in college we were attending a practical in histology, the study of tissues and cells in the body. After finishing the assigned task we were having an easy moment and generally lazing around. We did not realize that some of the professors kept a very keen vigil on what is going on around them. One of my friends in his curiosity plucked a hair from his head and started examining it under the microscope. He did not realize that the professor had caught him at it. Our beloved professor was an ex-army officer and a strict disciplinarian, so we were generally in awe of him. He immediately shouted and called my friend to the head table. My friend was trembling and feared the worst as he slowly started moving towards the head table. There were senior professors there including the former army officer. One of the other professors was in a recumbent posture on the chair as if sleeping. My friend got a mouthful and all he could do was apologize profusely; he was completely terrorized. After a fifteen-minute lecture and a warning my friend was asked to go back to his seat. As he was crossing the seemingly slumberous professor, who had until then seemed oblivious of the goings-on, the latter suddenly asked my friend a question. My friend was sweating and fumbled for an answer but the entire lab started laughing after those tense minutes. The professor asked my friend rather innocently, "Kahan ka baal tha?" (To which part of the body did the hair belong?). Despite the anguish, the agony and the distress the professor's query enlivened the proceedings, and dissipated the tension. Drama and tension become a part of the doctor's life. To alleviate these things it is imperative that a doctor is witty, jovial and cracks jokes.

An anecdote which explains what happens when smart patients outwit smart doctors comes to mind. A patient with a sexually transmitted disease went to a renowned doctor. The diagnosis was very apparent, the case looked grossly neglected, and the doctor was very short-tempered at seeing such an irresponsible patient. He shouted at the patient and asked him where he had gone before coming to him. The doctor asked this question as he thought that he was the first consultant. The patient very innocently said that he had gone to Dr Mrs. XYZ for medical consultation. It so happened that Mrs. XYZ was our doctor's wife! The innocent reply led to a great deal of embarrassment. The reaction of the doctor this time was blushing and flushing on the face.

Another joke comes to mind. A neurosurgeon friend was frantically running after a patient. On being asked why, he replied that it was the third time that the patient got a haircut at his expense with the promise that he would get operated on. The haircut happened but the operation remained a dream, for the third time running! The collective reaction from the fraternity was, "Thank God the patient did not have a urological or a gynaecological problem!"

AUTUMN LEAF: THE PREFACE

The autumn leaf symbolizes age, maturity, experience, strength, and above all the capacity to face adversities. Needless to say, if the leaf has reached this stage of its existence and is still clinging to its base, it has to have the qualities mentioned above. Any active professional, like the clinging autumn leaf, goes through a lot of experiences, several ups and downs. Many authors have written about their experiences in their respective fields. Some write without having experienced what they are writing about. Fortunately, in my case I am saved from such a problem. I have gone through the mill as a doctor and have witnessed the pros and cons of being a doctor; have been a witness to the ethics and the un-ethics of it all, and have the requisite gall to comment on it. I fully believe that one has to be wary while dealing with such matters. There is a minuscule minority of readers that reads whatever is placed before it for knowledge and information. There are others who take everything at face value, still others who are skeptical about every point they read and understand – and finally there are those who do not understand at all, but go with the tide. But a book of this nature belongs to a class of its own. Here a professional tells his part of the story! Does his part of the story hold water? Is he justified in writing such a book? If a retired general or spy writes a book, readers will lap it up. But what about a book on doctors and the medical profession, written by a practicing surgeon?

My profession has ceased to be "he hems sawbones" as described by Charles Dickens. The advances in medicine are such that some operations can be performed with the aid of laser – a minimally invasive technique. But what about the human side of the profession? Has it kept pace with such advances? Do we have sanctity in our professional lives? Do we knowingly mislead those who do not know what we know? Does the professional get away with it all because everything has several answers and multiple angles? In our country does a professional own up to being illusory and not call it fortuitous? Is it safe to own up in an emotionally charged country like ours, even in the medical field?

Things have come to such a pass that, according to the mortified masses, one profession which is slowly but surely turning decadent in our country is the noble profession of healing. I belong to the medical fraternity, therefore I thought of writing this book. It seeks to answer broadly all the questions that arise in a person's mind. This book is not meant to ruffle feathers. The story has its moments of sarcastic wit laced with a bit of serious introspection. The book is all about becoming a doctor and leading a doctor's life. It also deals with the reasons why a few good professionals change somewhere along the way. Is it society which precipitates the change? Is the exploitation by or of the patients? Is it greed and competition with other unconnected professions? Can medicine be categorized as a profession where earning is according to man-days and the level of investment? If the statement 'take your fees but do not be greedy' is to be accepted, then who defines what is the correct fee? Unfortunately the governing bodies cannot. The governing bodies are entangled in their own issues.

When I chose to become a doctor, I was fulfilling my parents' dream of having a doctor from the family. Did I want to become a doctor? At seventeen years the answer to this question was confusing: yes and no. My immaturity when it came to making the decision and my naïve nature were the reasons. A no would have been a likelier decision, but a few ostentatious scenarios shown by the people who mattered swung the decision to a yes. Therefore this is a book about doctors by a practicing doctor who honestly did not want to be a doctor. Strange, isn't it?

Being an emotional person I do things with a lot of passion. After I decided to become a doctor, I did not let any diversion or setback come in my way. Though I was fond of internal medicine and gynaecology, the aura and glamour of surgery attracted me towards doing my post-graduation in that subject. Medical practice became a passion. To excel and be the best was my motto. However initially I could not achieve what I aspired to. I realized that brilliance in one's subject, honesty and hard work need not translate into success always. I reckoned that a keen business acumen, glaring display and braggadocio were equally important characteristics for accomplishment. The intensity that I lived my work life with therefore needed expression. This expression was not forthcoming through any other forum. This book was written to express that perturbation. Not surprising that this book has formed inside me for many years now.

Medical education was fun and the ten years spent in the hostel were superb! The relations with teachers were excellent and the level of education and quality of professors was world class. A few who were not very expressive or intelligent made up for their deficiency by working hard. We had original and ingenious ways to trouble the less fortunate. Our batch was good in academics, sports, extracurricular activities and "Dhamaal". Our synchronous tapping of the wooden floor of the lecture hall was a way which went down well with juniors for many years. This was our way of conveying that we did not want to study that day. The parliamentarians can copy this method which is nonviolent and very effective. It was only when I stepped out in the real world that I realized I was unfit to be a doctor. Still, I hung in there till success came and now I have memories which I want to share with you.

When I started this book two years ago, there was a certain amount of anger, frustration and remorse in me. It was more to do with my not achieving success as I saw it in my mind's eye. I had dismissed my life, considering it wasted. I used to go through the mundane routine, with the growing feeling that I had been left behind in my profession. I was losing my willpower and just did not have the wherewithal or the inclination to learn anything new. The past haunted me and weighed me down perpetually. I believed I had had a successful past as per what I wanted, when I worked in the hotel industry, before enrolling for medical studies. While experiencing my disillusionment with the medical world, I could only think of other professions and the successful people of those professions. I knew that life was a war fought everyday. I also knew that only the fittest survived. Fitness is both physical and mental. I plunged into all the ways possible to make fast money. Met the major players in my line of work. I offered them professional sharing and even renamed the sharing as follow-up charges, just to soothe my conscience. The flow of patients increased. I was pleased and thought of going across for support to more doctors. After the initial burst, references started drying up. I could not understand the reason behind the declining quantum of work. I thought of many reasons, including the misgiving that I may not be competent to give the required or expected results through my medical skills. A thought that I was an outsider in my own country just because I spoke another language (albeit an Indian one) made me consider relocating to North India. In this period the restless mind got attracted to the unknown. Several astrologers, pandits, soothsayers, tarot card readers, hand readers and the like benefited. Pooja to cleanse the body and mind and rituals to drive away evil were offered with a lot of fervour and in the belief that things would get better. I started sporting favourable gems and stones – my hands looked like the treasury of an erstwhile maharaja. Pilgrimages were undertaken to increase the inflow of patients. All this yielded nothing but loss of revenue, added expenditure and more frustration. The mighty Lord and the unknown power were evidently busy elsewhere.

Slowly but surely the patients started coming back without references, and through my moral strength I started regaining mental composure. O sing praise to the Lord for He is good! The anger on self, which was an outcome of the frustration when I started writing this book, dissipated. My angst gave way to a rational analysis of all that actually went wrong while the Lord was busy! A lopsided, unprofessional tirade filled with hatred and venom started softening and became more balanced. I decided that I had to survive – how could I let go and allow the disparities to persist? I was angry not because my practice was not booming, or because I was not earning millions like the others in my profession. My anger had to do with issues of right and wrong. It was a dilemma then and even today, though things have changed. I am not the loser that I was on the way to becoming, at the ripe old age of 45 – as they say, life begins at 40, and mine had just begun too! And it is too precious for one to just let go.

I now know that I have the conscientious strength and courage to do what I must. A comparison with others does not perturb me anymore and takes a backseat in my scheme of things. I believe in what I can achieve. My wife, well-wishers and my bad weather friends, the soothsayers, astrologers and tarot readers all helped me get out of this phase and predicted and pushed me into going ahead with this book.

The title and contents of the book underwent several changes. From a strong tirade against my own fraternity, in which I did not spare even myself, it gradually grew into a more evolved, sober and balanced piece of serious thinking based on the idea that if any decay has set in, then we need to acknowledge collective responsibility – society, the governance machinery, the socioeconomic milieu, the increasingly competitive medical industry, all have contributed to the way things are. It is a multitude of complex problems. Our social fabric, our beliefs and our illiteracy have together led us to this pass in more ways than one. It is interesting to recall that in the early eighties there was a major social campaign in Delhi. The campaign slogan was not to marry your daughter off to a doctor. Everybody was asked not to marry off their daughter to a doctor. The authors of that campaign were doctors themselves and the awareness message was to show the stark reality that even after hard work the remuneration to most doctors was pathetic. Since then we have come a long way into the new millennium, but the competition has become worse, and the income gap seems only to have widened. The most educated are never the most affluent.

I still need to assess my achievements. Have I achieved what I had set out to do? What I intended to do was to spark off introspection among the doctors and patients towards respecting each other's viewpoint. The medical profession fetches good money, and while it may not be the best, it is certainly an honourable profession and also adequate if one considers the respect attached to it. The appeal is not to make it a money-spinning machine at the cost of fellow human beings' sufferings. I could not have indulged in deeper analysis since it would have opened up a can of worms and would prove offensive – that is definitely not the idea. I know I have not answered many questions which crossed my mind when I was in a state of despondency. The reason being, I do not want to negate the good work being done by the medical fraternity by harping on what is not being done. In fact, the absolute motive is to put forward an argument for a smarter, healthier, more fruitful doctor-patient relationship. I hope to kindle a thought process. If it helps anyone, I would consider my mission accomplished. Then, a sequel is always there. A good and appreciated work may bring out the author in me. I am an incurable optimist! And why not? Without hope, life will have no meaning. A Wrong Prescription can be corrected and made into a Right Prescription or a Follow up Prescription. I wish you the best of reading and I hope you shall enjoy it, just as I enjoyed writing it.

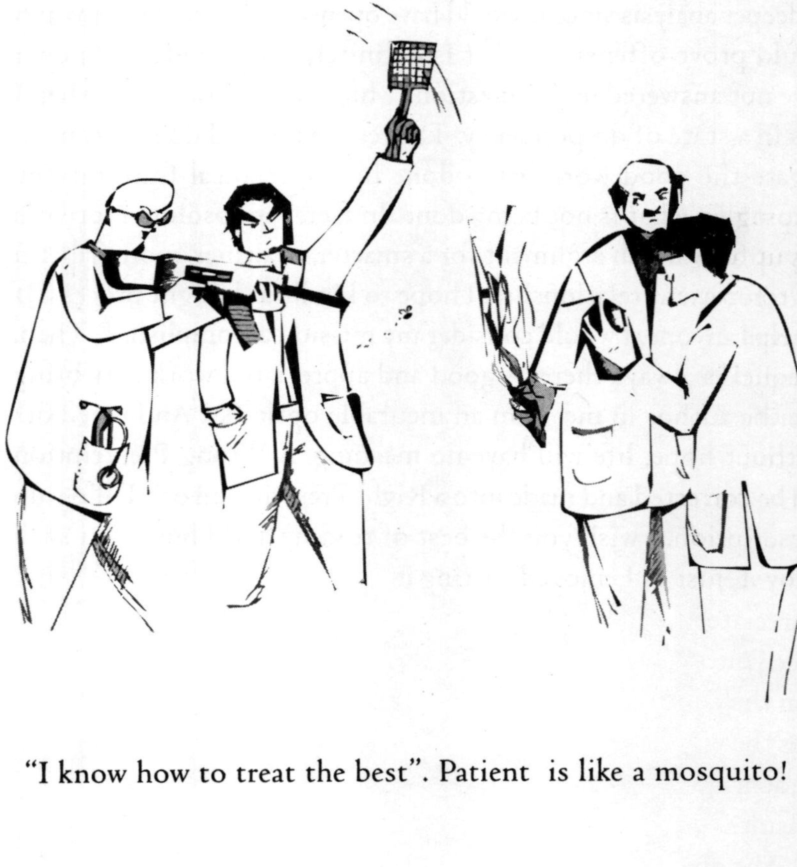

"I know how to treat the best". Patient is like a mosquito!

CHOOSE YOUR DOCTOR!

Almost all my colleagues have at least one non-medical friend who calls up at any odd hour and asks for medical advice. It is always to fill in for some other doctor who attends to him/her but who is not available at the moment. Usually the call is for an ailment which a medical intern can handle. No slight to the interns, as their theoretical cognizance is excellent. In the initial days when socializing was the high point of my day, everyday, whenever I received any such calls, the response was sincere. The thought was that the friend's health depended on my sincere and thorough guidance. However, experience has taught me that free counsel is least appreciated and rarely acknowledged. The pedestal on which you place yourself while rendering advice is taken into account rather than the advice itself. As all subjects undergo metamorphosis, so does the way to admonish. When I receive a similar call now, I ask a prudent question like, "What kind of a doctor would you like to consult?"

The directory of doctors is akin to a ready reckoner of famous gourmet outlets. There are four types of eating outlets. At the top of the category come the ones which serve the best food and are famous because of that. The second category consists of the ones which are famous because of their marketing and business skills and not necessarily the cuisine or the taste or the food they offer. The third category comprises the ones which serve fantastic cuisine and are authentic in taste but are not famous, and the fourth category is the ones which neither serve good food nor are famous. Choose what your taste buds allow.

Doctors can be classified in the same way. Take your pick. If you can get and afford those who are famous and also good, you are lucky. And if you get any of the other three categories without knowing, God be with you. To put it any other way would be a travesty of the truth. How can someone be famous and yet not have quality? Elementary, my dear Watson, as Sherlock Holmes would have put it. The second category qualifies for this reputation, since they are known for all the wrong reasons. They are the most thoroughbred PROFESSIONALS. A tongue in cheek description would be to say that such people spell 'professional' as PRO-FUSS-I-ON ALL. Little real wisdom but a barrage of apparently profound verbiage on the smallest and simplest of issues. 'PRO' in their spelling means precisely what it does otherwise in the world, 'public relations officer', 'FUSS' stands for self-aggrandizement, 'I' is self-explanatory and 'ON-ALL' is the gullible world. The secret of success therefore is a thrust on I within the framework of PRO activities for all.

It is worth visiting all the different categories and seeing the different ways all these pros tackle the same problem. I have created a linkage with my first profession, namely hospitality, and would love to share it with you. After all, we are in the same business, the doctor and the hotelier, namely that of servicing customers. The request and the rejection run something like this: Appointments please converted into the hotel jargon. The first and second categories will be the most difficult to approach. We are booked! No tables (time) in the dining hall (consulting room), we apologize! Only if you are very hungry (seriously ill), shall an assistant see you! Why did you fall sick (hungry) before making a booking with me? Do you have a reference from a VIP (a reference made by an MAS (Mutual Admiration Society)? Has a VVIP recommended you (the ruling type you know!)? Shall not allow you to peep in my premises, sorry! Please do not try to find out that I have time! The patient, Mr. Ill still perseveres! The third and the fourth category need to be identified first and that in itself could be a herculean task. The patients find out on their own accidentally or friends and relatives are forthcoming. Their long-term experiences help them decide whether a doctor is in the third or the fourth category. Both the latter categories are low profile, do not have a strong reference base and are not known in the conferences, media, or medical promotional activities. Often even the competing peers do not consider them as threats. The medical representatives do not speak about them and generally the staff members in a hospital stay away from them, when it comes to showing relatives and friends for medical problems. It is necessary to highlight here that all the patients may not agree to this categorization and may not adhere to the definition unanimously. It is always based on individual experiences. All doctors do not treat all patients successfully all the time. Let us begin with the first category. See you post-consultation!

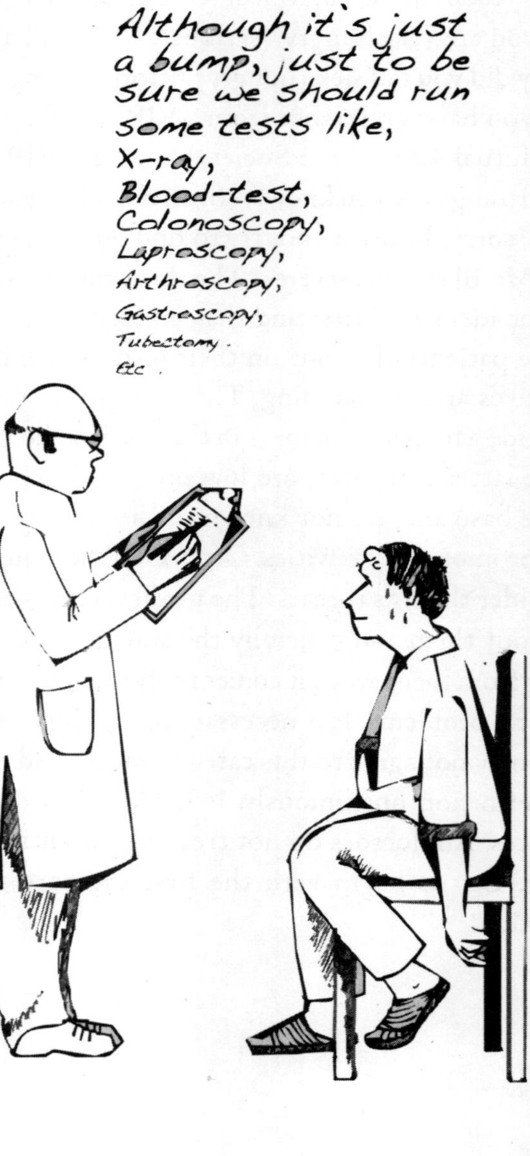
Although it's just a bump, just to be sure we should run some tests like,
X-ray,
Blood-test,
Colonoscopy,
Laproscopy,
Arthroscopy,
Gastroscopy,
Tubectomy.
Etc.

CATCHING THE DOCTOR'S EYE

The saga continues. With great effort, a category one doctor is reached. The first and the greatest hurdle is to convince the receptionist that the patient merits THE DOCTOR'S kind but immediate attention. A questionnaire, more elaborate than the tax declaration form, is orally answered.

This is how the conversation goes thereafter with the receptionist:-

After the customary name, age, sex, etc. symptoms of the ailment are sought.

One recalls the Gujarati saying and mumbles "cha karta kitli garam" ('teapot warmer than the tea'–in other words, the assistant seems to be throwing his weight around and claiming a greater importance for himself than for the doctor).

However, answers have to be provided.

The moment you say that you have a pain in the stool passage area, the Admin Assistant asks rather innocently if a visit of or to the taxman has recently happened, or if multiple visits to government departments have happened, or if any other doctor especially the likes of a proctologist or urologist, have examined.☺☺☺

After asking the accompanying contingent to step back, he nonchalantly but firmly asks in hushed tones about sexual perversions.

Quite cheeky! What is the relevance, one asks?

My 'sahib' talks to friends on the phone and mentions these as the foremost causes of this tormenting pain which afflicts a lot of patients.

Thank God I do not have an 'ass-is – constant' in my office!

After this exchange of information, the advice follows, which ranges from diet to medication and lifestyle.

Finally the 'ass is-constant' arranges an instant audience with his boss.

A sudden stroke of luck befalls.

But the mind wonders - what more will the boss add?

The only comforting thought being that if the employee is so "enlightened", how would the boss be!

The accompanying task force is asked to wait outside. This could be a major cause of mental turmoil to a weak patient when he is entering the doctor's den. A few close ones in the task force probably know more of the commode habits than the afflicted himself. Wonder how that happens!

On request to the boss a self-styled leader is permitted to enter.

Wow!Intimidator or tactical supporter?

'Namaskar' Mr. Ill. I have seen your file. Please step inside the examining room. Mr Assistant, remove his clothes and ask him to assume position.

The harried mind wants to ask, "Sir, please ask me what my problem is?" The mind echoes again and again.

Is there democracy in the medical field or fascism, dictatorship!

Like a puppet the body succumbs to the order. No explanation as to what is happening or going to happen.

Target shooting!

Cannon ball practice!

Please take deep breaths. Some ointment applied.

Aaaah! A finger poked in?

The best possible plausible thing. Could it be something else!

Though the intensity of pain increases, the cold sweat is due to the vivid hypothesis, following the jab.

Please wear your clothes and come out. Please sit and my junior consultant will explain things to you.

Once again the agonizing wait starts. How is it that the one who puts the masala and salt is not the one who tastes! Can the dish be prepared correctly? The silly mind ponders again.

The junior consultant arrives. Mr. Ill, you are suffering from F.I.of A and possibly also H.P.P. Besides these, C.D.D. cannot be ruled out. Your DRE is very classical. A conservative treatment plan can be worked out but not before you get thoroughly and totally investigated.

By whom?

The C.I.A. and F.B.I., with the local C.B. initiating the inquest! One mumbles.

Pathological and radiological investigation! Thank God.

A differential diagnosis may emerge. We then may contemplate surgery. Surgery though the last resort is the most definitive and in my experience the best and the most logical final option. Only in case you want to undergo an uncertain conservative medical regimen, would a treatment option other than surgery be considered. We have already told you up front that the non-surgical option is always there. We believe in honesty while dealing with all the patients.

Any questions?

The little courage that was there is ebbing away, and Mr. Ill hesitates to ask whether the anatomical part in question is a hardened criminal. Is the part only to be investigated radiologically or to be investigated under POTA also? The sheer awe created by the doctor is mesmerizing. The "task force representative" nevertheless displays valour of sorts. The only words that come out are, "What investigations?"

Gleefully, the junior consultant says, thinking that the surgical option has been accepted: All pathological blood tests which should include the functioning of the liver, heart, lungs and kidney. These are from the anaesthetist's viewpoint. There are other viewpoints also, so some logical and some neurological tests are to be done. From the press and consumer court angle illogical, philosophical, classical. The strongest accompanying relative gets a sense of attrition, "Whatever you say, Sir", since the name and aura have preceded the meeting. A crushed patient fearfully asks whether a conservative regimen can be tried. "Oh sure! This is the prescription. The receptionist will tell you how to take the medicines."

By then the contingent has made friends with the receptionist. On receiving the file, he does a great job of explaining how to take the medicines and how to follow instructions. He gives his contact number. He also takes extra care to convince all present that the boss is the best and that the boss is always right.

A second opinion is definitely warranted. Somebody please help!

The category two doctor's evaluation is a must. Let us see how he fares. Let me tell you he is second only in name, so carry on, Mr. Ill.

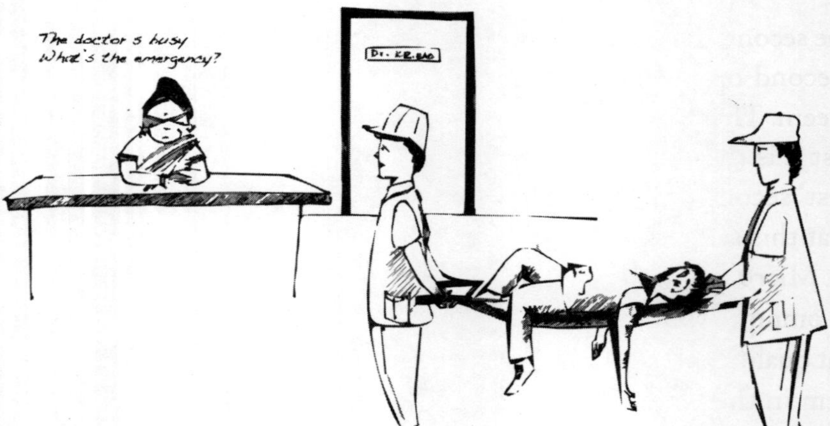
The doctor s busy
What's the emergancy?

SECOND AMONG THE BEST!

The second opinion has to be from one among the best. It is called a second opinion, but this second doc is never 'second' in self-esteem. The doc's mindset is that if there is a something before a first it is this 'second'. How to give shape, size and breath to this 'first' second and prove that there is something before the first is what this second doctor is all about.

Micro-organisms, God, and this second category of doctors are omnipresent. Mind you, for them it is in fact the first category that qualifies them. Only naïve and frivolous minds like ours group them in the second category. A recall of their name should be a reflex action and not a thinking exercise. For the ill-informed, an uncalled for, irrelevant and illogical question comes to mind. Where and how do we find them? The question and the answer is difficult enough to be included in the TV show, "Who Becomes a Millionaire".

If the question is asked on the show, then the options would be

a) media face
b) hoardings and advertisements
c) all of the above,
d) none of the above.

It does not take a genius to guess the correct answer. It is "C", as the only choice of the answer. If one still has doubts, an audience poll will settle it.

A further evaluation by an investigating mind may reveal a commonality and a pattern, of this 'first-first' / 'second-first' category. We do not intend any pun, and hara-kiri of a kind is being committed, but the characteristics have to be mentioned because of the research that has gone in to establish this community. The inclusion criteria are

Normally have a background of getting admitted without having to go through the rigors of medical admission. A trust seat, a donation seat and abnormal-door entries for a degree are pretty much found in everyone. Generally but not always, not a first-generation doctor. They have their mentors, parents or somebody in a high place. Only then the crowning takes place. Another profession of our country, politics, comes to mind because of the hold of dynasties on that profession. Why blame only a few!

A prominent feature found consistently is that any media-related event, or any event of mass recognition will have a member of this category presiding over sessions. The session could be medical, non-medical; social, anti-social, etc. The bona fides of the chairman are neither age-related, nor experience-related, and never knowledge-related. They are as the saying goes "God's own dung." These larger than life heroes are Superman, Batman, Spiderman and Plasticman, rolled in to one.

The theorem that 0 comes before 1, is challenged and redundant in these cases. '0' is derogatory, and 1st has been taken up. ½ and ¾ are incomplete and anything raised to the power after 1 is actually complementing 1. Thus to prove a point and to discard the earlier theorem, 1 is not raised to a power, it is the power which is raised to 1. The power that is raised comes before the 1 and is not 0. In conclusion, this connotes a lot of 'bull' to mathematicians, but the category we are talking about is different. It is trendy and unparalleled and has a singular unique identity.

If further probing is done, a very classical observation vindicates this category. At an age when hundreds of medical graduates and postgraduates are entering the field and are at a struggling stage, our young friends occupy the most expensive, up-market piece of real estate. They start their practice from this place, amid swanky interiors, luxurious settings, immaculate surroundings, and a good number of patients seeking opinion and treatment. Though they are spared the rigours of admission to the medical field and hard work during the student days, knowledge is not a casualty. Medical insights are at a D.N.A. level, therefore the right to occupy a prime position at the medical social podium becomes a birthright.

After identifying them, the experience that the same patient shares vis-à-vis his pain in the anal region is something like this: The experience is heavenly and definitely heady. Heavenly not for the feeling or the ultimate experience, but owing to the fact that everything that happens goes above the head. In trendier linguistic parlance it is called overhead transmission.

A call for an appointment receives answers from busy to unavailable. Though a patient hardly ever asks for reasons of non-availability, reasons are always given. The principal reasons are that they are chairing a session at a conference. Normal attendance as a delegate is not for them. Another reason given is 'patient visit'. Now this is valid for all doctors, or so one thinks. Sure, but these visits are never in the city where they practice. A study tour or a stint as visiting faculty somewhere normally completes the list. To a few more enlightened people, who understand this business, presenting papers is a solid and legitimate excuse to show the paucity of time. However, when the patient shows inclination of going elsewhere, an appointment is promptly given.

The ambience on entering the premises leaves one breathless. The way the employees carry themselves is impressive. Had they not been caused by a nagging ailment, the patient's trivial ills would have been treated and would have become all right by merely entering the gorgeous place. Nonetheless the appointment has to be gone through, so carry on Mr. Patient.

"Do you have a pain in your anus?" is the question asked. Before an answer is given, a profound statement is made. "In my vast career, (which by any account is not more than two or three years), I have treated thousands of such patients."

"Wow!" you feel.

"I have treated the royal family, the first political family, the biggest industrialist, the most well-known sports personality, etc."

This guy is great. He has put my anus alongside the royal and celebrity class. At least my anus and I are in that league owing to my disease. What a refreshing thought. But the damn pain has not gone! It persists.

The focus is lost due to this feeling of grandeur, and many claims to fame get diluted However, statistically, how could a person have attended to so many patients in the short career and still reside somewhere else? Imagine and calculate, treating thousands of patients in two or three years. The driving distances and freshening routines would themselves have taken a considerable part of that time. Even if a person resides in the anus, he cannot complete thousands of treatments in two or three years. His success means: no vacation, no food. It is still a possibility because super humans are at work.

On examining, these were the exotic thoughts:

"...My experience suggests that your ailment has already been diagnosed and investigated. I have a protocol of my own which I delivered at the Universal Congress on Anusitis, but your earlier doctor has already stamped a diagnosis. I can differ, but in the ethics of practice, I cannot show it. Therefore let me just treat you. You require an early operation immediately. Medicines have no role. Only those who do not know the art of surgery depend upon medicines. I have travelled across the world, and treated thousands of patients! My laptop and PC have all the data. See for yourself the kind of work that I have been doing ..."

One wonders how this ailment was being treated before this guy was born.

"...I shall operate on you with the latest technology and modality. I have done hands-on training with Dr. Prof. Havcreatedduffs. He is the pioneer of this technique and I was lucky to be associated with him. He is from the Nevrheard University School of Anal Sciences in the USSA. It is in Foolsville, Bragasmuch, Assakissus, USSA. Very authentic and credible, one would think. A huge effort to establish credibility.

Before you can show your innocent ignorance, the Doc is at it again.

"...Aha, I knew you were familiar with the world trends. This new technique does not require any cuts or stitches, and it is painless. You shall be out of the hospital faster than you came in ...."

The Indian patient is the best, because he does not ask many questions. Not even the relevant ones. Still, in a stuttering voice the patient asked how many patients had been the victims of the modern surgery before him. Not in those words of course.

"...We have a follow-up of ten patients in three years. All the patients are absolutely fine. Two out of the 10 died after 6 months due to age- related, normal factors. Three were re-operated for minor complaints. One has not shown up and only one has some pain which is minor enough, and is controlled with pain killers. The other two who were operated by Dr Havecreatedduffs are doing well ..."

"Sir, your hands-on experience has paid rich dividends. Either the professor was holding your hands or you were holding the patient's hands. What a pity that I can't actually say this to you."

"Sir, any side-effects of this new modality?" is a genuine question which a patient has a right to ask.

"....With the kind of training I have, the vast travel in various countries, the local, national and international conferences that I have attended, the papers that I have presented, the series of 10 patients, one of the largest coming out of Foolsville, Assakissus, I can emphatically declare that the new technique has no side-effects. The anus being a central part, how can side-effects take place? The effects are all central ..."

"Sir, why is this technique not commonly known or advocated?"

"...Mr. Anuspain, when Archimedes, Galileo and Einstein presented their visionary work, it was not accepted. Everybody cannot afford the new technique and my friends cannot go for hands-on training abroad. Jealousy and professional rivalry are small but significant reasons. I have professional ethics, so I wouldn't like to comment any further ..."

"Sir, any common references that I can relate to?"

"...You want to talk to the CM or what? Here, talk to Mr. Buffoon, the tycoon. I have his private number."

"Sir, the private number is okay, but would he talk about his private part?"

"...Nothing is private for a doctor, Mr. Anuspain. Besides, Mr. Buffoon talks to me on a daily basis, without paying my fees. His private part and the operation are behaving erratically after the economic crisis..."

"Sir, please do not call him, just tell me the expenses of the operation."

"...Do you have any health insurance that can allow you cashless transactions? All new things are costly, for reasons we are all aware of. Though my charges are on the higher side, I shall honour you by giving you a special concession. You are showing a lot of faith in me. I am a considerate man, you know. Since you do not have a health insurance policy, I cannot charge you much. My routine charges for this operation for non-health insurance patients are Rs 13 lakhs, but for you I shall charge only 12.75 lakhs."

"What! If that is routine and reasonable, then what is on the higher side? Sir, please excuse me, I shall come back later."

"...Why, what happened? ..."

"Sir, my part is not worth that much. My pain has suddenly disappeared on hearing your fees. If I quote your charges to my family, they will all become your patients."

"....I can give you a further discount ...."

"Sir, I am cured by just being in your august company and do not think that I require any further treatment."

"...If you feel that August is not acceptable to you, I can reschedule our meeting for September! That is after my return from Australia. I am going there for Annual Ass Ailment Congress."

Please CARRY ON DOCTOR.

THE BODY REBELS

After a mind-boggling session with the best and the righteous, the ailing part has started fearing the obvious. The part says, "enough", the heart says "let it rest", the mind says "there has to be a cure" and the brain says "go in for another consultation". If our Creator had endowed each part with individuality, a civil war of sorts would have occurred. Since the brain has become the anus and the heart has started emitting gas with the mind throwing the filth out and the anus ruling the brain, it is turmoil of the most exemplary kind. The body becomes like a small boat in the ocean. The waves are tossing it around and this time the "advisor" sends the person and his body to someone who is not very well-known but is supposed to be very competent. Where, one would think, might a professional of this kind be found? Dial yellow pages! Even Sherlock Holmes could not have found one such. To start from a retired or a senior professor of a teaching institute is the best bet. Even if the line of specialization or faculty is different, reference from a good student may prove to be sufficient.

Finally a reference is found.

Sir, I am calling for an appointment. I am Ill Anuspain Dungsting. I would like to see you since I am suffering from a very state of the art disease. I believe it is a disease which doesn't respond to conservative treatment, and therefore requires a high-tech operation.

"...Mr. Dungsting, you can see me at your convenience. I am available from 10 am to 1 pm and from 6 to 8 pm, except on Sundays. You need not take an appointment. You can walk in and shall be examined within 20 minutes at the most. In case I am stuck elsewhere I shall give you a call and let you know of the change in the appointment..."

"Sir, your address please?"

The pickled brain is already having doubts about the credibility of his advisors' advice to visit this category of doctors.

"...How can a doctor have time ?

How can a doctor be so courteous?

If he is good, why is he not arrogant?

Is it humility or marketing gimmick! Is he worth visiting?"

Hail the pondering pickled anus-ed brain taking a call on a person and personality based on telephonic salutations!

"...I practice in People's Society, off Humanity Highway. My nursing home is on the first floor of a commercial complex called Peace of Mind Plaza. You will have to take the staircase which is located behind the complex. It is in the eastern suburb of the city ..."

"Sir, I shall be there on Monday."

A reluctant yet affirmative mind mechanically responds.

Hereafter the deluge begins – the heart, the part and the fart all shout, "No way!" The reason has more to do with fatigue of travelling to the other side of the city and then climbing the stairs to reach the venue of a practitioner who has doubtful credentials. Obviously the mind revolts and the first meeting is ducked.

The mind becomes a recluse. It does not utter a word to the other parts. After seeing the grief and the sorrow of the mind, the rest of the parts relent. The creator has not bestowed individuality to any of them. A second call for re-appointment (though with a sense of sheepishness) is in order and is therefore planned. Since emotional reasons are the best excuses for our emotional society, something emotive had to be created, otherwise the so called doctor could feel bad. The options are to kill somebody on paper and in the mind, for no wrongdoing of that soul, or to make a non-medical yet a social tragedy, which cannot be investigated by the doctor.

Sir, I am Dungsting. I had an appointment with you but could not come, because my wife's sister's husband's nephew, who stays in Timbuktu, ran away with a street wench. My wife got upset and fainted because she was trying to get him married to her kitty party friend's brother's wife's niece. I had to go home to attend to her. As I was to come to you from my office I had to forgo the appointment. Can you please reschedule?

"...You can walk in at any time", is the answer for the second time as well. All the body parts unanimously accept that the doctor is indeed polite and not short-tempered. Thank God for small mercies!

In an uncoordinated effort, the body reaches the venue in a few pieces. The mind is what the eyes tell it to be. A very modest set-up. No secretary! A ward boy performing multiple roles! No waiting patient in the lobby! Is it the right place? Suddenly the bell rings and a patient, obviously from the People's Society, steps out and as if in a relay race, gestures that I can walk in.

"Sir, I am Dungsting."

"...What ails you?"

"Sir, I have a pain in the area around the anus which gets worse when I sit for long."

"...Is the pain related to your bowel movements? Do you have constipation?"

Aha! The first relevant question in the last fifteen days, I think.

"No sir it is not. The comparison sheet opens up in the mind and suddenly the brain leaves the anus and reaches where it should have been all along. The ailing part starts getting restless, as if to show where the affliction is, and the heart settles down into a relaxed mode. What a difference the approach of this doctor has made to the body. But then I am one of a kind. Most people like the categories that I have already visited.

"...Have you changed your job recently or perhaps changed the chair you normally sit on?"

"Yes. I have changed both." Elementary but how true! Suddenly the diagnosis is at a striking distance.

"...Is the surface you sit on very hard?"

"Yes. Earlier I had a thick cushion, and now I sit on a piece of wood, that too for longer hours."

"...Examining you is not necessary but a casual look will do. Please lie down on the couch and we shall get it over with in a few seconds. I need not even do a finger examination and no internal examination is required. Your pain is purely muscular due to prolonged sitting on a hard surface. A pain killer is required only if your discomfort does not go after you get yourself a thick cushion. Come back to me if the discomfort continues after seven days of using the cushion..."

"That's it? No chills, pills or thrills?"

"...Sure. Why? Do you expect something more serious?"

"Sir, please have a look at these files, the advice and the recommendations."

"...There is nothing for me to comment on. A case comes to mind which shall explain everything to you. The only thing is that he came to me when it was too late. Medicine is a tough, demanding profession, but God has created a machine which has an in-built auto-healing processes. The human race is older than modern or even documented traditional medicine. Patients survived then and will continue to survive and live. The ratios and the percentages are the raging debate which, if settled, could render a lot of things redundant. Medicine still remains an art in applied common sense while treating most ailments. The moment we leave reasoning and correlation out and start applying modern technological advances, we get trapped in misdiagnosing. A clinical diagnosis is followed by technology to prove that we are on the right track. After diagnosing correctly, the treatment modality may vary from conservative through wildly flamboyant to utterly nonsensical ..."

"Sir, you were telling me about a case...?"

"...Yes. I remember this case in which the sharp minds of several peers used all possible modalities to diagnose an ailment in which, had common sense been applied, the patient would have benefited more. They used an AK-47 to kill a fly rather than something lighter like a plastic spatula. Patients of that kind become vivid memories..."

"...He had pain in the scrotum and testes, which increased as the day progressed. He was treated for multiple infections. All the treatments were less to do with conviction, more a matter of shooting in the dark. He was investigated left, right and center with USG, CAT, PAT, VAT and the like. When there was no end to his misery, he approached one of my colleagues, who had returned from abroad. Thinking that the latest advice and devices would be available, he went to him. Prior to that he had been to many psychiatrists as well. Clinicians thought his brain had been balled, and the poor guy got it extricated from there. He finally realized that his problem was not functional and had there been a pain meter it would have reflected his suffering. The friend who had returned from abroad recommended a diagnostic scrotoscopy. It is still to be researched, but if a person has come from abroad and has a scope, he has to use it. Under anaesthesia, he distended the scrotum with gas and put in a scope. He found nothing abnormal and ended the procedure. This unlucky patient was in severe agony because his scrotum had become a balloon. It took him many days to recover from this trauma. However he was led to believe that he must go and show it to a scrotologist. When asked what a scrotologist does, he was told that this is a super-specialty branch emerging across the western world and they deal with only that part of the human body..."

"...The western world had the developing world's part symbolically and now physically!"

"...This frustrated patient went to the so-called scrotologist who had been a keen observer for 6 months. During his observership in this field, God only knows how many scrotums he must have examined as the western world does not allow observers to touch any part. He must have observed pretty paramedics, and brushed his own scrotum on a daily basis and several times. That's the only way he must have completed 6 months in scrotology ..."

What hogwash! There is no branch of this kind.

"...Nevertheless the hapless and helpless patient went there and got himself examined. Dr Scroto gave him the alarming advice that he get himself castrated. Yet it appealed to the patient as he was sick, tired, frustrated and depressed. He went back to the scrotoscopist and asked him to remove the pearls. It was the saddest day in the history of medicine.

"...The scrotoscopist did a laparoscopic removal. He told the patient that this was the first case of its kind and that an article would be written about it. Nobody had done a laparoscopic removal by the minimally invasive keyhole route. The patient got discharged on the fifth day after surgery and the doctor gave him a certificate which advised six weeks of rest from work. He naturally paid through his nose for the surgery done...."

What is the use of keyhole surgery in our country if the patient requires 6 weeks of rest anyway?

Perhaps the fact that it is painless!

This reason is never covered in any journal.

"...The article must have got published. The patient lost interest in the follow-up procedure as his ailment resurfaced after six weeks of rest. Ultimately he came to me on the recommendation of one of my own patients. I asked him what he had done while he was resting for six weeks. He said he was in just his 'lungi' and nothing else. I concluded that the problem was not in the scrotum or the testes or indeed any other part of his body. I told him to stop wearing his tight underwear and his pain would go. Lo and behold! The patient got cured of his ailment and to this day he repents having gone to the scrotoscopist. He pledged himself as my goodwill ambassador..."

Getting back to the original issue of choosing the right doctor to consult, this one was an amazing experience and having recovered with this doctor's advice the patient thanked him profusely. The doctor made him understand that all that glitters is not gold.

The implication of not understanding the ailment in a patient but recommending treatment options can be disastrous for the patient. This is more so if the results are negative. It is not without a reason that teachers tell us to use newer modalities only after the froth has settled.

I remember having learnt a few things this way while I was doing my post-graduation. Since I was still coming to terms with the local language, conversing with and understanding the patients was difficult at times.

A few hilarious incidents happened but not at the cost of the patients' health. My colleague and I, being the junior-most in our batch had to sit outside in the verandah most of the time. We were responsible for sorting the patients according to their ailments and sending them to the seniors inside. It so happened that in one of those OPDs, it was very crowded and we were trying to work our way through as efficiently as we could. One of the patients walked up and I heard him saying only the word "kapasi". In my enthusiasm I told the patient in broken Gujarati that he was on leave. We had a senior Dr. Kapasi, who was not present that day. Without carefully evaluating what the patient was saying, I went on telling him that the person he wanted was absent. The patient kept on saying "kapasi" and I kept on saying "nathee". This lasted till my colleague got involved and he started laughing. He interpreted and told me that the patient was trying to tell us that he has a health problem - he was complaining that he was suffering from warts or a callosity. He did not, as I had thought, want to see Dr Kapasi.

A similar episode happened when I was working in the ward. I was doing the paperwork and carrying out orders relating to the morning rounds. A patient's relative came and complained, "Sahib, kharchoo baoo thay che", meaning that the patient was having loose motions. Being essentially a Hindi-speaking doctor, I understood her words to mean "... it is very expensive or the expenditure is very high." I gently told the relative that, since it was a major surgery some expenditure was inevitable and that we would try to keep it to the minimum necessary. The relative went back looking totally disoriented. God only knows what she must have understood. After thirty minutes she returned and told me the same thing. Again with a lot of composure I explained the same thing. In another fifteen minutes she returned with the same complaint. This time I got a bit curt, but before I could be rude the nurse in the ward started laughing. I looked at the nurse sternly and asked her not to laugh at this serious matter. She got up and gave some medicine to the relative and explained something to her. After she left, the nurse told me that the patient was complaining about loose motions and not about money! I sure did look silly then! I was lucky that no damage was done. A little knowledge is a dangerous thing and the fourth category of doctors in particular bears witness to this fact. Yet, for the sake of adventure, it would be a good idea to try out the last category. Considering the fact that the ailment has gone, the naughty mind and not the knotty mind shall go in for this exhilarating experience of listening to the ones who are neither famous nor competent. So carry on Mr Anuspain!

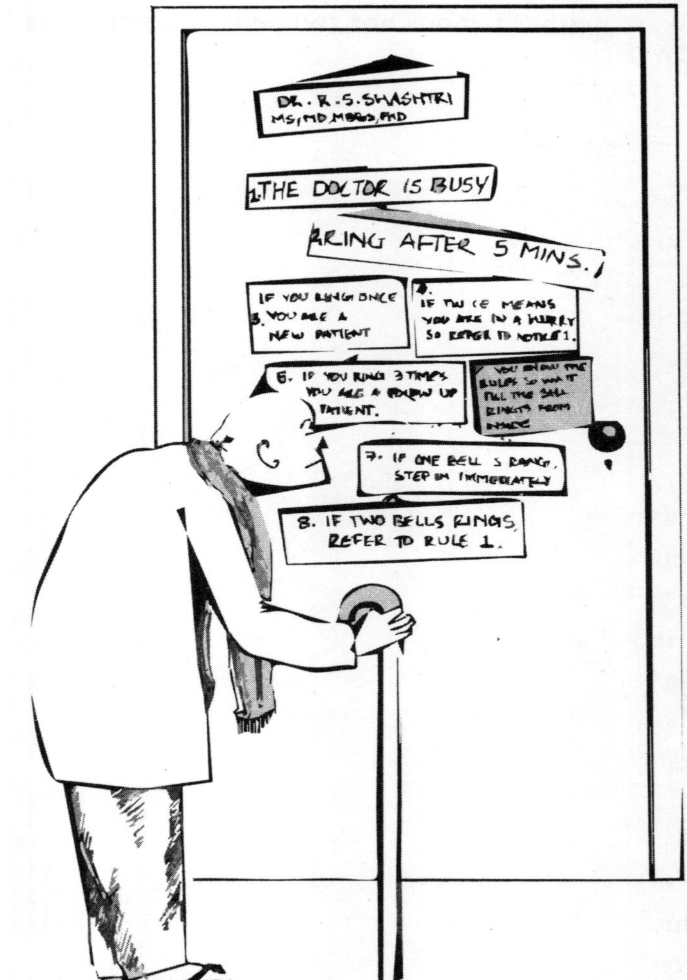
DR. R. S. SHASHTRI
MS, MD, MBBS, PHD
1. THE DOCTOR IS BUSY
2. RING AFTER 5 MINS.
IF YOU RING ONCE
3. YOU ARE A
NEW PATIENT
4.
IF TWICE MEANS
YOU ARE IN A HURRY
SO REFER TO NOTICE 1.
5. IF YOU RING 3 TIMES
YOU ARE A FOLLOW UP
PATIENT.
7. IF ONE BELL S RANG,
STEP IN IMMEDIATELY
8. IF TWO BELLS RINGS,
REFER TO RULE 1.

A MIRACLE ALL THE SAME

We all believe in miracles and usually hold God responsible for them. But I witnessed a manmade miracle. From a patient who moved around as Ill Anuspain Dungsting, he is finally back to his normal self. He was named after a bum cleansing ceremony in childhood as A.P. Dun. He was forgotten because the friends renamed the initials Anuspain Dungsting, owing to the ailment.

After going in for boxers under his formals, (he was so paranoid after hearing about the case of the tight underpants and the wooden chair), he also opted for a thick cushion for his office chair. He felt as if he were sitting on a throne and keeping an eye on everybody, as he became the tallest one among those seated ... who knows, he may qualify for a different kind of job. Internal security, for instance!

One should not care and feel embarrassed at sitting or doing a thing which can cure his insides and that is security of the best kind. After sitting like that, he felt like securing legal protection for his petite buttocks. Just a few weeks prior to this he would have traded them for anything in this world. That's what I call a miracle!

After getting totally cured, the naughty self in Mr. Dun and his 50 kg perfect frame cried out for the final category doctor's consultation. Again the search began, but nobody in the fraternity of 'med-i-call' told him about this category. He had no clue how to go about it, till his friend's ten year old son told him that students who failed many times over can never be successful even if they get into professional colleges. The child has to be respected for his advice but in a real life scenario, most things depend on the business acumen of an individual and how he takes advantage of the situation to optimize his gains. There are multiple examples in the medical field of doctors who were ordinary, or poor in their performance while doing the course, but are revered as the best doctors a city can boast. As the search was leading nowhere, a visit to the medical college administration department by Mr. Dun yielded a few names. One of the names, that of a well- known doctor who had been in the past a president of RAMSE. was a startling revelation. The word 'RAMSE', stands for Repeaters Association of Medical Students Everywhere. To qualify as a president, one has to have failed five times during the medical training program. However, for a reason Mr. A P Dun stayed away from selecting a post holder of RAMSE, as that is a success in itself, and went for a guy who had seven trials (though not of the judicial kind – 'trial' here is the colloquial term used for repeating the medical semester or year). He did not feel the need to call him up and just set off towards his location in the far flung periphery, beyond the city limits.

The premises presented a primitive look with a wooden bench outside. Mr. Dun had forgotten his cushion so did not sit as the bum was far more precious than anything else in the current scheme of things. He observed a wonderful innovation, brilliant for his kind of thought process. In the waiting area was a bell with instructions on how to use it which read something like this:

1. The doctor is always busy.
2. After waiting for five minutes please ring the bell.
3. If you ring once, it means you are a new patient. If you ring twice, it means you are in a hurry, therefore refer to rule one.You may use the bathroom if the need is too pressing.
4. If you ring three times that means you are a follow-up patient. You know the rules so you know how long to sit. 5. A bell will ring from the inside. If you hear one bell that means you can step in immediately, but if you hear two bells then refer to rule one.

Curiosity got the better of him. Precisely what this doctor was busy doing was the mystery he wanted to solve. He peeped in and saw the doctor reclining on an easy chair with his legs propped up and listening to something because only head phones could be seen. Mr. Dun realized the reason for being busy was genuine, but he could not fathom how the bell could be heard when the ears are plugged. Nevertheless having come this far he wanted to try his luck. He rang the bell once. Did not get a response. Rang the bell twice not necessarily remembering the rules. Yet no response. His despondency increased. Rang the bell like a maniac and to his horror the doctor ran outside. One could see the anguish on the doctor's face. Before, Mr. Dun could say anything, the doctor shouted that these many bells were for the fire drill. A plausible explanation for his alarmed and hurried exit from the cabin. Mr. Dun naturally apologized, unable to tell him that he had peeped in.

The doctor made him sit on a wooden chair. Mr. Dun was horrified but had no choice.

He just wanted to get out of this Dr. Bell's clinic (named after the bell) as soon as possible. "...What are you suffering from?", asked the doctor. Before Mr. Dun could finish answering, the doctor asked him to show him his tongue. After giving a cursory look and telling that the tongue was healthy, he started writing something. Correlation please, someone: what did anal pain have to do with the tongue? After a few minutes of silence Dun was asked to show his tongue again. On his complying, the next comment was even more intriguing and true to a certain extent, though irrelevant to the current disease.

"The tongue is the mirror to the ailments in the body", the doctor declared emphatically.

"Sir, I have a pain in the anal area and there are no digestion complaints."

He ignored this statement. The naughty Mr. Dun was asked to turn around and stand. He was repenting the adventure that he invited on himself, but did what was asked of him. With a small hammer-like instrument the doctor hit the patient's elbow and biceps and buttocks and asked him to sit and struck his knee joint and ankle. Then he poked his underfoot as if trying to draw a boomerang. The toes widened. After that he asked Dun to close his eyes and checked the skin for sensations. Your reflexes are giving erratic, uncoordinated, nonsensical responses.

Mr. Dun could appreciate it all.

At the end of what seemed to Dun like carpentry work, tapping as if to hammer a nail, the busy doc concluded that the local part was misbehaving and was not under the control of the high command. Mr. Dun was told that "The high command sits far away and it gives a command to the local ass, to behave in a certain way, but the local ass who is supposed to be in command, refuses to take orders from anybody else. This discrepancy leads to friction between the local ass and the high command and the anal area which is the local representative of the larger ass takes the brunt of this command problem and that is the reason for the discomfort. I can understand your agony because that is what happens in our country...."

Till that time Mr. Dun was totally lost in the change of commands and the commanding highs and lows, flabbergasted at the most illogical but nonetheless impressive knowledge and explanation of the disease. Had this not been the last of a series of consultations, he would have fallen for this commanding interpretation.

"Treatment, sir!" he pleaded.

"...One of the commanders has to be brought into sync with the others..."

'Diplomacy or force' was the focus of the next question.

"...There are hard options and soft options. The soft options are wearing cushioned pants, not sitting at all, going to the bathroom once in seven days so that the renegade ass does not strain the local commander, sleeping on water beds..."

"What are the hard options?" Dun naturally had to ask.

"...The hard options are complicated neurological surgery. We can start with electroconvulsive therapy for the highest commander so that national fiefdom gets jolted into submission, followed by neural dichotomies at the spinal level for treating the regional commander and his renegade ass..."

"What shall we achieve ultimately?" That was the last question as Mr. Dun was awestruck, perplexed and totally hypnotized by this "analibanisation" of the laden kind, on the SWATY area, having the distinction of being a geographically important area of his body.

"...You would not have any pain, or any other sensation for that matter. The mutiny of the commanders would be crushed, and all will fall in place because the importance of the ass and local commander will go away. There would not be any control of the high command and the high command will be very weak due to multiple collisions (coalitions) of different modalities of treatment..."

"Any side effects, sir?" was a reflex question.

You may permanently lose control of your motion sensors and motion. Adult diapers are available in the market, but nobody can cure your pain better than this. You have come to me for a problem and I have sorted out the problem amicably. Your pain shall disappear. Please do not worry yourself regarding the side affects.

Mr. Dun walked out after paying whatever was asked for. Did not stop even to collect the paper on which the commander-in-chief was writing something. On his way back he was recollecting with horror the war zone through which his mind had wandered.

He could not stop pondering on the other bigger question. What happens to all the other patients who can be influenced and are gullible? He took solace in the thought that the real Commander-In-Chief, who is invisible and watching everyone from up above, is the final authority; he is the one who dictates life and death and suffering. Hail that power! Mr. Dun stopped at the nearest temple to pay his obeisance.

There is a million dollar question which comes to mind. Where does the training and knowledge that is essential and has to be brushed up on frequently come from? After graduation and a few years of practice, when the doctors get busy, is there time dedicated to upgradation of knowledge? Is it from books or continued medical education or some other teaching aids? One sure would like to know!

KNOWLEDGE UPGRADATION

Patients are the best teachers. A doctor has to spend time in the wards during the medical course to get the most out of it. There is a hierarchy within the ward and that ensures learning in a systematic way. The junior-most is the one who records the history of the patient's ailment. He is the closest to the patient till his junior enrolls under him. It is a yearlong learning period. Though considered clerical work, it is in the long run the most rewarding. All successful clinicians are first excellent history takers. The clinical findings and later on the pathological tests and diagnosis depend on how well the junior-most presents facts to the seniors. Above the juniors in first year, there are students of the second year and then the registrar who presents the round to the head of the unit. This ensures that the patient evaluation is very minute and thorough. Next in hierarchy are the students who have finished three years and have written exams too. The Senior Registrar is a doctor who has cleared his surgery exams but is still pursuing tenure in the government hospital. Above him, the Assistant Professor, Pool Officer, Associate Professor and head of unit (again a senior Professor) complete the team / ministry. This jumbo Cabinet is a constant phenomenon in most teaching colleges across India. Knowledge and learning begin here. An incident which took place when I was in the college and was in the second year of my Master's:

I was in my fourth term and had juniors and seniors below and above me. A sixty year old man with his two official wives came to the hospital and was admitted in the ward for prostate enlargement, which was causing difficulty in passing urine. He had been taken through a digital rectal examination (DRE) by the boss in the OPD. Admission was out of the question without the boss clearing it in the OPD. The junior-most took down the patient's medical history in the ward, examined the patient and wrote the notes. He did a digital rectal examination, in which a finger is inserted in the anus to evaluate the local area. That is the only clinical way to evaluate the prostate. He was unable to evaluate the pathology. When his senior, a second year student of surgery walked in, this junior requested him to evaluate. This was the protocol. The second year student did give his opinion but was not very certain. In came the registrar who was requested to do a DRE as it was an interesting case. The registrar obliged. Every doctor who walked in was asked to do an evaluation as it was an interesting case. None of us realized that this was not very amusing for the patient and his two wives. All of them were getting restless and apprehensive. The examination was then done also by the senior registrar, pool officer, assistant professor, associate professor (total of seven or eight). All of us started waiting for the boss to arrive for the post emergency round. After the round got over and the patients who required examination in private were lined up, this old man started shouting. He was asked to pipe down by the ward staff but would not listen. The boss called the old man first and asked him what was bothering him. The old man asked to be discharged. When the boss asked the reason, he replied very agitatedly, that if the treatment for his ailment is inserting fingers then he can have it done at home. Why should he waste his time coming to the hospital. Though the patient was pacified then, it certainly was a lesson learnt. A hands-on teaching program for the undergraduates was therefore cancelled.

This patient would have run away or filed a case for perverted manhandling, had he been fingered by a batch of twenty more students!

Reading medical books, referring to journals and attending clinics during the curriculum is mandatory. After all one has to clear the final hurdle – the exam for the Master's Degree. Some of us secure a Doctorate after the Master's course.

The medical curriculum that we are subjected to is so saturated and theory oriented that correlating all this learning with actual illnesses observed in patients takes a long time. The confidence level of fresh medical graduates is not too great, and that of novitiate surgeons is even lower. It is like knowing that a pain liniment relieves the pain, but not knowing the area or the reason of pain. Then knowledge erosion sets in and if ways of refreshing the mind and brain are not found, early decay sets in. That is why knowledge upgradation after leaving the institute is very important.

Correlation between the theoretical and the practical makes a doctor complete. Intelligence in a doctor is reflected by this key phenomenon. If common sense alone is applied and no attempt is made to correlate symptoms with theory or vice-versa, this backfires, as it happened in one of the undergraduate exams. In a medical college in North India, five international students were appearing for their physiology exam. The first who went in was asked about the temperature regulation center in the human body. His answer was the tongue and as expected, he was asked to leave. His rationale was that when dogs need to cool down they stick their tongues out, so the same is applicable to humans. He was sent to the dogs.

The second candidate walked in and was asked the same question. He replied, "It is the kidneys". The explanation being that urine gets concentrated in hot weather and flows freely in cold conditions.

He too was eased out.

The third student went in and was asked whether all the candidates coming in were friends.

"Buddies", was his answer. "It shows", was the examiner's comment. "...Since you guys are friends and are quite alike, let me ask you the same question, to find out which of you is the smartest.

"....What is the temperature regulating center of the body?"

Very confidently this student replied that it was the skin.

"...Not bad", said the examiner. "...You are on the right track, but the center is called something else. Incidentally why is it the skin?"

"...Sir, it is because when we feel hot, we sweat from the skin and when it is cold, we get goose pimples. As far as your second part, I do not know where the center is...."

Finally the last of the friends was called in. This fellow couldn't speak English well but he looked promising.

"...What is the temperature regulating center called? ..."

"Hypothalamus", was the correct answer given and the professors were overjoyed, especially the internal examiner.

"Bravo!" and "Excellent!" were the encouraging remarks given. "...You seem to be the smartest in this group."

"Where in the body is the hypothalamus situated?"

With the newly found confidence, this guy replied at the top of his voice:

"...Testes, sir ..."

"...Get out!" was the frustrated response from the professor.

"...But before you go, I must know why you think it is situated in the testes?"

"...Sir, when it is cold the testes move up and when it is hot the testes move down."

It took the friends several years to clear the undergraduate exam.

There may be stray examples of students who are not intellectually adept and who get admitted to medical colleges. The above students were thankfully not from India. As mentioned earlier, medical education is a highly saturated course in our country and the quality of education gets compromised owing to the non-availability of basic aids and the load on teachers, especially on the clinical side. The professors have to manage the vast numbers of patients that reach the government hospitals and teach as well. A few changes and an increase in the number of teachers may help. The onus of finding alternative sources for improving knowledge lies on the individual and that's why the following 'parallels' who also impart knowledge are important.

The first alternative set of gurus is the pharmaceutical industry medical representatives – the ubiquitous MRs that we, as independent consultants preening in our own cocoons, encounter while trying to brush up our knowledge and learn about new molecules and drugs.

The focus of the pharmaceutical industry, as of all industry categories, is definitely growth and profits. As with all companies or organizations, the pharmaceutical companies are also multinational, national, local or unknown. The kinds of people who represent these companies to us doctors immediately inform us about the kind of company we are dealing with. A new company with fewer resources will not mind putting a novice into the field. A multinational or a nationally-based company will normally grill their personnel and choose the best available from the lot. These men deserve far more respect than they get. Doctors do not consider their inputs very valuable. The higher the platform in practice, the less the time given. Meeting someone to learn something new is, alas, not usually the prime concern. Yes, if there is a business offer, anybody is allowed, otherwise a select few are given preference. Personal likes and dislikes do matter but ulterior motives tend to govern the decision regarding meeting (or not meeting) people. Of course, every job is to be respected and anybody who does a sincere job and puts in diligent work is appreciated. Everyone has their own flaws and limitations and we all learn to recognize and live with them.

Take the case of a new MR walking into a clinic or hospital. He initially falters in the salutations and then recites and reads from the visual aid. His nervousness is apparent. At times the coordination and statement of purpose is so poor that the briefing is done to the wrong target audience. At other times the product highlighted is not relevant to the core practice of the doctor. When the representative is abruptly interrupted, it is obviously followed by a profuse apology. It should be admitted that a multinational and national company official knows more about certain molecules and drugs than the doctors themselves who profess to treat patients. Yet to establish and prove their supremacy the attitude of the doctors is to allocate very little time. All hell breaks loose if the rep crosses the limit by asking certain pointed questions. When a technical expert accompanies the marketing representative, his technical knowledge of the molecule is definitely better and superior to that of the doctor, but showing it causes casualties in prescription. One medical representative asked a certain doctor which type of bacteria was afflicting his patient. This was in a routine discussion about antibiotics and efficacy. The doctor got agitated, perceiving this question as a challenge to his knowledge of microorganisms. He threw the representative out. These power games between representatives and doctors often turn self-destructive for the representatives. The doctors may engage in a vendetta by not prescribing the products the offending representatives advertise. Therefore successful representatives who are good at marketing choose to be diplomatic. They never commit this kind of "hara-kiri". "Never challenge a doctor" is their mantra; the doctors win the power game, the representatives get their medicines prescribed!

Gujarat has the privilege of being home to prominent pharmaceutical companies which have a pan-India footprint. This includes some of the multinationals. This means that doctors are well targeted, and can often begin to feel wanted, if just because of the number of sales representatives that visit them. As Samarpan Hospital's practice grew in stature especially after its renovation and expansion in 2008 we suddenly began to feel that we were in the big league. The reason was the sudden increase in the number of companies who wanted their share of the prescriptions. We were getting popular! While the companies targeting us rose fourfold, we waited for a commensurate increase in patient inflow!

In much the same way as teachers are evaluated by their teaching prowess, MRs are always evaluated on how they impart education. From walking in to the chamber of a consultant to imparting knowledge, the evaluation of the MR can be categorized as good, bad or atrocious. There are a few very good ones too. Actually all of them are in a Catch 22 situation. They have to evaluate a doctor in a split second and impart knowledge according to his mood, the time given and the quantum of knowledge that their company has asked them to convey. If the rep walks in when the doctor's mood is foul, or the doctor's knowledge is in question, and his assessment of the situation is proper, he realizes this instantly and chooses the path of a quick and a quiet exit. If he walks in when the doctor's mood is jovial, he is encouraged to complete the visit despite his shaky knowledge of the subject. The really atrocious reps are the ones who continue to recite nursery rhymes even after multiple visits. They walk in and read the visual aid as if they were reciting. Such rote recitation often spoils the doctor's mood. Good reps teach doctors about the molecule, its pharmacology, its powers, its side effects and the indications for using it. The marketing guys are very reticent about the side effects of a molecule. They try to avoid any adverse comment till a new more advanced molecule of the same family of medicines is launched. The older molecule is dumped because it had limitations, they then venture to say. Fortunately, in our country, the patients' resilience with regard to bacteria or any other intrusive element is so good that the old molecules still work wonderfully well.

The professional approach of any MR can be compared to Indian classical music and the various ragas. Some of them put the doctor to sleep while others wake him up. Some tend to become very friendly and some remain cold. To learn from the tranquilizing variety is marginally better than trying to squeeze milk out of a bull. To say that no knowledge is attained would be a dishonest statement: daily prescription knowledge is somehow attained in spite of difficult conditions and soporific MRs.

The second source of knowledge is none other than our own pharmaceutical industry sponsored CME (Continuing Medical Education) courses and conferences. In earlier days there used to be a season for holding these CME courses and conferences. Now, learning jaunts are organized throughout the year. While there is no end to learning and it can happen anywhere and anytime, the efficacy of any learning program increases manifold if the effort to organize and share knowledge and information is optimized. Conferences are a good means to share lessons and have a dialogue between the industry and doctors, but both should do their homework before attending these conferences. Without this, conferences do not fulfill their learning potential, instead often turning into wasteful marketing events.

To begin with conferences are not always conducted only with a learning objective. Commercial motives are now accepted as valid for conducting conferences. Speakers at the conferences are often invited based on their potential to give future business to the inviting company. Even if one accepts that commercial objectives are the order of the day, and non-negotiable, one still hopes that conference discussions will contribute to a doctor's ability to deal with real life situations. Sadly, often the application of theoretical learning to actual practice is missing too. In this scenario, one questions the sustainability of new theoretical advances that are claimed. These advances benefit the peers who are attached to medical institutes which have a mass patient base. What about doctors who do not have a state of the art parallel paramedical or clinical diagnostic branch set up? The vast majority of doctors, therefore, remain outside the purview of advances in the field of medicine. Conference discussions often cover the latest breakthroughs in medicine and specialization in the developed world and metropolitan cities. State of the art knowledge is necessary to understand the extent of treatment one can suggest or prescribe. But what cannot be done, especially in emerging markets, is applying that knowledge in day-to-day clinical practice, owing to infrastructural and expertise constraints.

This implies that conference interactions are either social events for medical networking or well-disguised platforms for launching doctors or medicines, promoting pharmaceutical companies or all of these. Delegates carry memories of the conferences. The success of a conference is based on the food served, entertainment and facilities. Scientific content is never a strong point of discussion. Serious learners do accept the take home message from dignified speakers. Where and how to use this message is the impediment.

It is fun to attend these phenomenal gatherings and be amongst the august doctors of India. Given that the season to attend national conferences is November through February, 'august' in august sounds funny, but august in other months is fine. For the rest of the year there is a halo of knowledge shining radiantly behind the salt and pepper hair of a doctor or the full moon of his bald head.

Knowledge without application is more frustrating and counterproductive than ignorance. This knowledge is like reading the books and not going to the wards for clinical application. How can one learn medicine without actual patients?

Often, Indian medical students choose a medical school in another country as their final school of learning. Often this is under someone who is unknown in India. He or she may be known in their own country. These doctors hope to acquire their competitive edge through international education, which is largely likely to be through observation rather than practice. They then return, trumpeting the need for compartmentalization and specialization. In other words, the message is "call me or send me the patient". The exploitation of brethren has not got a sadder and a more classical example. Often, a graduate doctor holds on to a patient as long as he possibly can at the risk of spoiling a case or delaying correct treatment unreasonably. A postgraduate doctor, even after realizing the limitations of his inputs at that stage, still clings on. Curing the patient is not the criterion because the expertise required is absent. Finally, the holder of a doctorate of medicine or surgery steps in, the super-specialist, and by then it is either too late for a normal recovery or a permanent cure is impossible. When all this happens inadvertently it is pardonable, but it is criminal if this happens knowingly. To this day this ambiguity is not being addressed in the medical profession, and this style of practice is not going to change. The legal experts have largely given the benefit of doubt to the doctors in our country.

However, holding on to patients where further expertise to handle their problems is questionable makes this situation prone to vacillation. There have been incidents where the doctor has referred the patient to a higher center and the patient has been cured totally, yet the doctor has been harassed and booked under deplorable sections. The complainant and law makers who connived should be reprimanded strictly.

How is the international faculty superior to our teachers? How our teachers with greater experience could possibly be superseded by rank outsiders is a point worthy of discussion. The systems of reporting are no doubt stronger and the ways of teaching more methodical in medical colleges abroad. The working conditions, the paramedical staff and the level of technological advancement are likewise superior. However, the inherent differences of race and environment, socioeconomic and traditional influences and tropical vs. non-tropical diseases make research and practice abroad completely different from what they are in India. So, can we justify learning there and practicing here? The workload on doctors here, whether in government hospitals, charitable and trust hospitals or even successful private consultation houses, is far more than in the developed world by virtue of our huge and ever-growing population. Worthwhile comparisons can only be made if such things as the average number of patients being examined, the kinds of diseases being treated, the socioeconomic and educational profile of the patient population, the infrastructural conditions of the medical system, the level of technology available and so on are at least basically similar. There is no reason to believe that our doctors are in any way inferior – they have more or less coped with the load, albeit in a constrained manner.

The flamboyance is missing in the system, just as the affluence and economic support is missing in the patients. This does not discredit the Indian medical hospitals and medical colleges, which continue to remain great learning places simply by virtue of the number of patients who visit and offer a doctor practical learning experience.

The Indian medical system does require huge changes and technological advancement and these should definitely be prioritized by the Planning Commission of India. Documenting a study and working only forty hours in a week on the clinical side will lead to an improvement in quality. If the same individual is asked to examine, in one week or a fortnight, the number of patients that he ordinarily sees in one or many years, quality will obviously suffer. This is the reason that Indian doctors are the best across the world – their powers of endurance are well-known. By comparison, when a doctor comes back to the realities of the Indian situation after observership abroad, it takes him a lot of time to adjust. Getting experience outside India is like sitting on a simulator and proclaiming that you are flying a 747.

I know a person who claims to be a teacher to the leading lawyers but does not have a law degree. He has seen court buildings only three times in his 70 years. He won one case owing to his great common sense and argumentative abilities. The only knowledge he gathers is from reading one newspaper daily. Yet his arrogance and claim to legal supremacy are unparalleled.

A workshop was organized during the days I was studying medicine, about 22 years ago. Medical academicians from abroad were invited to deliver the workshop. We learnt through the feedback that complaints of faulty infrastructure and inferior instruments were most common. Safeguarding patient interest was perhaps one trigger for those complaints, the other being that offence is the best defense. If something goes wrong, it is due to the setup (although, mind you, our Indian doctors manage to deliver results in all kinds of setups!). Anyhow, we were very excited to see the best in the world operate. We expected to learn a lot. What was found was that the foreign doctors performed dissections as well as our Indian bosses, the principles of surgery used by them were virtually identical, but their wastage of consumables was huge. Our entire month's supply of consumables was used up in the workshop where three surgeries were carried out. A country like ours can ill afford the luxury of such wastage. We would have conducted as many as thirty surgeries using the same amount of materials. It was encouraging to see that the patients got discharged in roughly the same number of days; they had the same complications and the same post-operative complaints as when we operated. No wonder Indian doctors do so well across the world! They are brought up under constraints, study with the simplest and the sketchiest of infrastructure and the weightiest of textbooks, and deliver services to patients from widely differing socioeconomic strata with amazing ease! So, when they get state of the art infrastructure and have the strength of knowledge already with them, they become famous!

Lastly but very interestingly is the case of multiple degrees which a doctor has to his name to prove that he is better qualified, educated, experienced and a thorough professional. It is the fellow and the degree one gets by payment of fees. The trend is growing and for every ailment a new society is being formed. Very soon a number of new degrees will join the ranks of FICA, FIAMIS and the like. Does a doctor require all these to prove that he is a better doctor than the others? Well, being a member is for his own good. Gradually degrees like FADRE (Fellow of Association of Digital Rectal Examination), FAPP (Fellow of the Association of Penile Problems), FARTS (Fellow of Association of Rectal Temperature Surfers), FWARTS (Fellow of Wishful Awareness of Ridiculous Techniques Society) will come into existence. At the end of it perhaps these will all be merged into one single association called FOFSI (Fellow of Fellowship Societies of India). Hopefully this would not happen. It should not and I am sure we take pride in our medical training and curriculum. So is there a real need for the cosmetic degrees? The doctor in society and society itself probably feel there is!

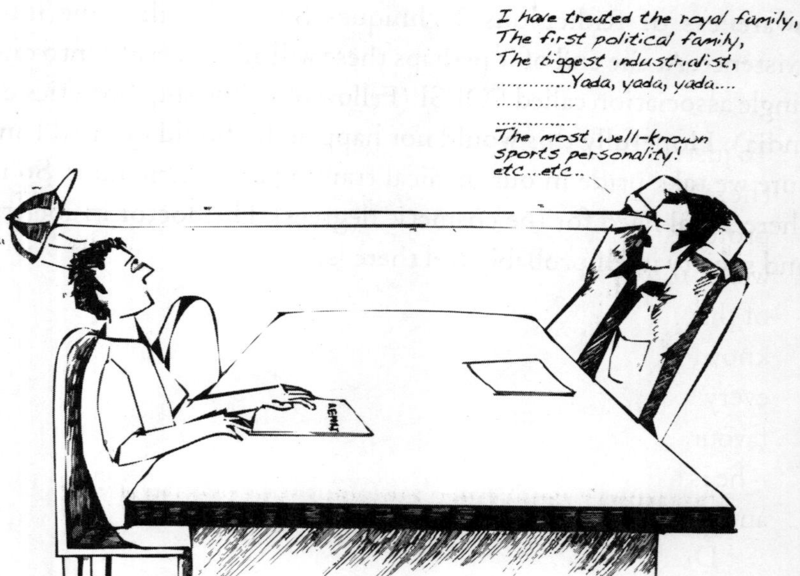
I have treated the royal family,
The first political family,
The biggest industrialist,
..............Yada, yada, yada....
....
....
The most well-known
sports personality!
etc...etc..

"Treatment by impressive C.V." Alas, for cure, patients need much more than just a talk.

DOCTOR IN SOCIETY

To justify his existence and establish his credibility, the doctor has therefore devised ways to overcome any doubts about his professional capabilities. The way he carries himself, the clothes he wears, the way he speaks and his air of inapproachability are all part of that façade. A necktie is a beautiful piece of attire which conveys knowledge. Even the body language and demeanour change with every patient; it's all part of learning how to project oneself favourably! A doctor in Indian society is a projection of an immortal – he is a hallowed man of God. There is one God inside the clinic; and there is another God above us.

Dress and address do matter in the world. But each has its place and time. Should the doctor be impeccably dressed? Yes if he is attending an evening party. Otherwise perhaps not, some may say. His business is to cure people and not waste his time dressing up. The healing business is a full time job. Healing followed by reading is the natural spread of time in a doctor's life. Refreshers for doctors are absolutely necessary to keep abreast of changes and advances in the research and development of the science of healing. Relationship management follows next. In fact successful doctor-patient relationships are directly proportionate to the amount of good work a doctor does in his profession. Dressing, though important, comes much later in the scheme of things. Moreover in a tropical country like ours, for the most part of the year, the weather is bound to be hot and sultry, and believe me I am not describing a 36-24-36 sunbathing on a beach. In this weather people of the developed world dress down to keep cool. We in our country are told that society likes to see a well-groomed doctor. He should have a trim and healthy physique. He should be very polite, humble and alert 24 hours a day for 365+2 days a year and should be available on call immediately. He should be a patient listener.

This is, of course, an ideal. It is like the budgetary projections of the Finance Minister which are famous for the stark variances between estimates and reality. This in no way implies that doctors are 'pseudo' personalities or hypocrites. Given a choice the simple folks will project simplicity. The question is not whether simplicity clicks or flamboyance. The question is whether true projection succeeds.

A wise man once said that the difference in the depth of knowledge between the best (knowledge-wise) and the worst is twenty-five percent. This is huge no doubt. The irony is that even the best know only seventy-five percent of the totality of medical knowledge. In the human body there is such an overlap between one faculty and another that diagnosing all the ailments in patients accurately is humanly impossible. That is why the brilliant are at seventy-five percent and the not-so-brilliant at fifty percent. The twenty-five per cent deficiency of knowledge is a mixture of unknown diseases, grey zones, faculty-driven jurisdictional restrictions and new diseases cropping up. To give an example, a simple stomach pain and vomiting could be due to a gastrointestinal problem, a cardiac problem, a neurological problem or a back problem. A single doctor may not have an awareness of all these ailments. Patients think (and indeed want to believe) that doctors are omniscient, but that is usually not the case. When a doctor who may be very knowledgeable asks for multiple tests, the same public, at least in our country, criticizes him for subjecting patients to unnecessary tests. This is probably due to two reasons: ignorance about the advances in medicine, and lack of finances. So what should the doctor do? As science unearths more and more discoveries, each medical branch has become more and more specialized, necessitating specialists to do full justice to the analysis of the ailment. There is no 'Harfan Maula', no 'Doctor Know-All' or 'Neem Hakeem' capable of instant and infallible diagnosis and prescription!

When I stepped into the field of practicing medicine, I never knew that all these things were more important than what you are best at. Besides the challenge it posed to my physical attributes, dressing up to go to work for a distance of 17 kms on a Yezdi 250 Classic, which by then was already ten years old, was not a strong stimulus for me. The other disincentive as far as getting dressed like a Peking duck was concerned was that while on the job everyone had to wear a uniform. It was during the entry and exit between the hospital gate and the fourth floor, where I practiced, that my finery was noticed, if at all.

My adipose-ly rich frame, with ordinary attire and a pair of either sandals or a 'mojdi', must have been horrifying to look at. I would have changed had somebody pointed this out to me, or had there been pretty dieticians or other good looking women around at work, or bariatric surgeons. Even the cardiac cases were not hyped. Not too many coroners were reporting natural cardiac deaths.

I just went on. A few genuine well wishers, including my beautiful wife, used to tell me that since I was a doctor I ought to look, walk and talk like one. The wife, who could have been the only agent for change did not press the point. The mission statement in my younger days was based upon an old saying to the effect that anything pleasurable in life is either immoral, or illegal, or fattening.

Having led a physically carefree doctor's existence with no regrets, I must answer a few questions on that score. Truly speaking the ideal type of doctor does not exist. Human beings have limited energy levels. Robots are now being used for creating that unlimited energy which makes them superior. Fashion designers are being roped in for robot clothing.

Do a doctor's looks matter more than his knowledge and his work ethics? Is it comfortable to work with the tied neck and caring more for the tie than the work in hand? Do we need a tie in our climate? We ape the west in such trivialities, while forgetting to follow the good things it has to offer. In the not so wild west, dressing up for work is the last priority of a professional, but working without hiding any thing from the patient is their forte. The belief in our wild east is quite the contrary and the explanation is that the society at large wants it that way. The quandary in a doctor's life in our country is not limited to attire. It is the volume of expectation of the public. Listing the amount of good that the doctors do will indicate a few things about a doctor's life, but the perplexing and frustrating side of their personality cannot be understood by the masses. However, I shall highlight in brief what a doctor's life entails.

The public, which expects the world of a doctor, changes its perspective and attitude when the time comes to reciprocate. If a person who has benefited from a doctor's treatment is asked for reciprocation, he goes out of his way to help. But what about a response to the doctors without knowing them. The call of duty for any doctor is of utmost importance always, or is expected to be so at any rate. In that context, the call of duty for any person who deals with public should be the same. Is that the case? Are ministers responsible? Is the bureaucracy answerable at odd hours? Is the engineer who constructed something which has fallen apart at 2 a.m., requisitioned to be there at that hour? Is it not an exercise in futility to try getting a valid and legal F.I.R lodged at the police station? If a request is made to a railway booking officer to book a ticket during recess hours or when he is shutting shop, does the booking officer agree? Noncompliance accompanied by abuses are the end result for such demands. Doctors do understand that unlike other professions, their profession calls for immediate response. If the car engine stops on a highway, a tow truck is pressed into service. However the engine with which the doctor's work should not stall ever. It is the life of another person which is at stake and once the engine stops, restarting it is impossible. There cannot be any comparison. Can anybody claim that they work on a running machine and can rectify it without having spare parts available?

Doctors do, and they show that the machine is on and even without spare parts, repairing is done. In this scenario if the machine does not get repaired optimally, the doctor is dragged to the court, he is harassed by the public and the media, and if, God forbid, the machine stalls, the doctor may well be arrested. Even if there is a complication which the doctor has rectified, an FIR of culpable homicide and wrong intention is filed. The law enforcers squeeze everything from the doctor and pose as if they are acting in the public interest. Instead of taking things head on, the doctor stumbles to protect his practice and image. In the case of any other professional taking wrong decisions or of a result not being as planned, everything is forgiven and forgotten. At the most, commissions of inquiry are formed. Such commissions invariably take a lifetime to give their verdict, and those verdicts are often of little meaning and use. A lot of public money has gone down the drain because of wrong decision making. Any action? Well, the only action is a few days of reporting, a bit of a public outcry and, if the opposition is active and alert, a few questions in the public legislature. Does any individual or institution actually end up paying for its wrongdoing? No way! But the doctor has to go on and put up with all this and more. In the process, the nobility of the profession suffers.

Only a few professionals get respect in our wild east. An I.R.S. officer, an I.P.S. officer an I.A.S officer and a politician are respected while in office. People even distantly connected to the above are automatically respected and their needs are attended to. 'Super quality, no complaints, pay (at a discount) when you can and it is fine if you cannot' is the attitude of the service provider. The political class demands these services, and no one dare refuse them when they are in power; likewise with civil servants. Every well dressed doctor wants to be in the good books of these people, and when they call upon his services, even a strike is not grounds for refusing, be it even for the most genuine of grievances. Guilt takes over, and though officially on strike, the doctors start running parallel OPDs. This is to gain public sympathy. Does any other branch indulge in this kind of hypocrisy? An engineer does not start to construct parallel roads or bridges while his colleagues are on strike. A banker does not start parallel banking services. Why then should the doctor? The debate is never-ending.

Legal provisions reinforce this compulsion on doctors to serve at all times. Such laws as ESMA make reporting for duty mandatory and that too with or without remuneration. One may not even question these laws. The doctors are supposed to be the noble guys. There is no need for food, clothing or housing for them. The reason is that the government gives subsidized medical education. All the basic rights of an individual are to be suspended in the case of doctors. Then there are other laws. It is mandatory if you are traveling in a car to stop and attend to a roadside emergency, especially if you have a doctor's sticker and a victim waves at you seeking help and asks you to stop. If the same car with a doctor's sticker asks to pass and reach an emergency when VIP blockades are put up on major routes without any information to the common man, then the doctor concerned is asked to stuff the sticker up 'the you-know-what'!

It would seem that in a crisis the doctor is a God, but when there is no crisis, the doctor is a fraud. If after treatment, the patient refuses to foot the bill, there is no law to prevent that. If an advance is asked for, doctors are vultures and if a bill is raised, they are compared to Don Corleone and the Mafia.

And God forbid if something unexpected happens, because then even the strongest helmet of ISI standards may not come in handy. Apart from the hospital bill, extra expenditure of real estate damage is to be handled and paid. To add to the misery, the media and the law start harassing the medical staff.

This lopsided equation between expectations and delivery is taking its toll. The gradual erosion of faith is due to this. Add to it the escalated establishment costs and the rising cost of quality technological aids. The project cost goes beyond the realm of economic viability.

Another interesting observation concerns an expectation of a different kind. A doctor falling ill is simply not on. He is treated as an outcast. He should never fall ill. The reason for indisposition is not important. It could have been the best restaurant of the town, where he had eaten the previous evening, or flu caught from one of the vast numbers of patients who come to him. The question asked at the first meeting after the information on his indisposition is, how can a doctor afford to fall sick? What the patient has in mind is that if the doctor cannot take care of himself, how will he treat others? The doctor looks at himself in the mirror after the question, expecting to see no image at all. After all, only gods do not fall sick and do not cast an image in the mirror. The rest are mortals. This theory is perplexing, to say the least. The doctor continues to ponder all this: after depriving medics of the right to "roti, kapda aur makaan", the right to fall sick is also being snatched away. And yet, the life of the professional doctor still has to go on.

But there is certainly a way out... the saving grace is that plausible lies are palatable to the public. The doctor concerned saves the day by saying that he was busy with an operation or was busy attending to a critically ill patient.

Just how plausible lies save the day in many situations is illustrated by this real episode. There was this young doctor who got a patient with a pain in the stomach. A clinical diagnosis was made and the patient was also subjected multiple tests. The tests and the clinical diagnosis did not match. The patient continued to complain of severe pain in the abdomen. The doctor advised an exploratory laparotomy. In this the abdomen is opened up to see if something has gone wrong inside. It is a procedure that was routinely deployed when the diagnostic armamentarium was not available. In remote areas patients still accept this rather than going to distant places to get diagnosed by complex machines and alien doctors. After the surgery and treatment the patient recovered. The irony of the entire episode happened after the patient was discharged. The doctor was taken to court because he came out of the operation theater and declared that the operation did not yield anything positive. He was ultimately spared by the court but thereafter he never tells the truth to the patients. He throws in a fair amount of dramatics while explaining, so that the patients and relatives feel that a lot has been done. This is done by exaggerating the problem as well as his role in curing the patient. The question is who made him that way?

A related set of difficulties arises from the fact that doctors are somehow expected to be far more abstemious and puritanical in their personal habits than the average person. The latter, when elated, may choose to get ethylated and sleep off the consequences the next day, but woe betide the doctor who does likewise. Similarly, we rarely think anything of a stick emitting nicotinic carbon monoxide vapours between the fingers of an acquaintance, but if that person is a medic, our eyebrows rise higher than the smoke from the cancer stick and the doctor's public rating descends in equal measure! It is only on certain bohemian festive occasions that we occasionally permit the poor fellow to partake of festive 'spirit' under the guise of 'prasad'.

Every body wants to be close to a highly successful and well-known doctor. One way of achieving this is what one might call the 'parasite posing as symbiote' approach. The would-be-parasite begins by bringing patients to the doctor and swelling his clientele. Pleased at this, the doctor becomes a buddy. That entitles the parasitic patient to walk in at any time. Though a crime for other patients, this is allowed by the doctor as he does not want to offend the friend who recommends patients. Nobody dare spoil a vote bank. Thereafter words like "I am like a family member of the doctor" are spread. Which side of the family, one may ask. The last thing in relativity is when the bills start getting tampered with and the patient's buddies have to be treated as VIP guests at lesser fees on credit! This becomes an additional headache for the doctor. How to treat this genre of patients is not taught in our medical colleges. This outstandings list swells and when the related sycophant is asked to muster up the 'moolah', a shocking reality bites. The one who had taken the responsibility of recovery suddenly starts shirking responsibility and the vote bank shrinks. Probably the relative has collected the money and used it, treating it as his commission. The relative in his new 'avatar' as tout casts his net afresh, scanning the list of ever gullible doctors. Doctors belonging to the top and the bottom rung of the medical fraternity are the usual victims. After a while, they catch on to the strategy, but by that time they have served their purpose and the parasite moves on to another unsuspecting host.

In our illustrious country, illiteracy is very high. Nonetheless when it comes to medical advice, almost everybody is a doctor and has a fund of self-proclaimed knowledge. The knowledge is not confined to allopathy, it covers homeopathy, ayurveda, unani, acupuncture, Chinese and Tibetan medicine. A lucky patient may come across an advisor who knows all of these. It is appalling at times to see scientific knowledge getting overruled by these "doctors", who have probably never even seen the gates of a medical college, leave alone reading the books.

That's how our wild East is. If a doctor advises something like an operation, then the sky comes crashing down. For the advising doctor, the wait begins because the patient has gone shopping to other doctors for alternatives to suit beliefs and pocket. Then it's explanation time. This time is not for questions which matter, like the side effects, the risks in surgery and so on. The obnoxious questions are such things as how long the surgery will last, what the patient would be permitted to eat, or when can the patient visit the bathroom.

The answers are given in monosyllables when the practitioner has been in the market for a long time, but in the initial phase of practice the effort is to please the important members of the family who accompany the patient. Speed is not really the concern for the relatives and it should not be, because an operation is not a Formula One race, but they probably calculate the number of hours that they will have to sit in attendance. A greater amount of time taken in the theatre is like a warning implying one of two things: one is that a complication may have arisen, and the second is that the doctor is stretching things to make a case for a larger payment subsequently. In either case it is the patients and the relatives who presume to teach the doctor what would have been optimal.

In what other field or vocation is the price tag of labour decided by everybody but the labourer himself? It is only in the great profession of medicine. Maximum exploitation, self-induced or externally induced and minimum reward. Please do not think of only the fifteen percent of doctors who are successful from every angle. What about the rest? Their reality is so different!

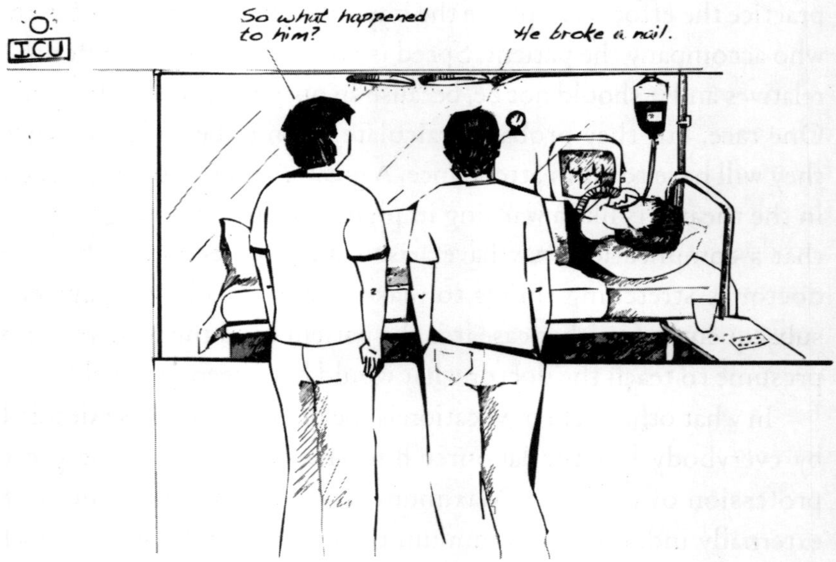
ICU
So what happened to him?
He broke a nail.

BUSINESS VERSUS ETHICS

Business versus ethics is a very touchy issue subject to many debates among people these days. The debate is equally relevant to the medical fraternity. There are two lobbies within the fraternity: the self-appointed custodians of medical ethics and governing bodies and doctors of the past era. The former would display ethics at least on paper, cite values of the medical profession and show that medicine is a noble profession and not a money making proposition. They have their arguments to substantiate their stand. Proving these arguments in public, especially among the patients, who have suffered and have been treated successfully or in patients who await treatment and are hopeful of a positive outcome is difficult and at times impossible. A book like the present one has not been written for the above purpose. However, there is growing disenchantment against the medical practice. The disgruntled people are increasing and introspection is required and here comes the need to prove the arguments in front of the most ardent supporters of the doctors. The doctors of olden days disapprove of what is happening now. Why and how this journey and thought process is changing slowly but surely is the moot point. The need to earn is there in every profession and every business. Today's world is fast-paced and everything is materialistic. There is no point in going into the analysis of what has brought about today's materialism, but the greed for luxury and the lust for earning a lot of money to feed that greed is driving sane people towards insanity – insanity purely in the context of rational thinking, not as a disease but as a thought process. But where is the line dividing the sane and the insane? What is wrong and what is right? Every thought process and treatment modality can have more than one option. To say that an option was chosen keeping money in mind is impossible to prove. The bubble bursts when something goes wrong. Had introspection been a stronger virtue, this situation would probably not have arisen. However there is a protocol which has been in place for a long time. It is not acceptable in today's world, but nobody can deny its existence. The Hippocratic Oath was written keeping in mind the nobility of the profession. The oath is taken by every person given the degree of medical doctor. The oath stresses three main things: the role of the teacher and his progeny, the role of the professional in practicing the art of his trade with social obligations, and the confidentiality of information relating to patients. It is probably the emphasis given to respect for teachers and to not indulging in wrongdoing in the profession which have suffered the maximum erosion. A few verses from the oath state:

"I swear by the almighty, that I will carry out, according to my ability and judgment, the oath and this covenant. To regard my teacher in this art as equal to my parents; to make him partner in my livelihood; and when he is in need of money, to share with him...

I will use treatment to help the sick according to my ability and judgment, but I will never use it to injure or wrong them." It goes on to say, "But in purity and in holiness I will guard my life and my art. Into whatsoever houses I enter, I will do so to help the sick, keeping myself free from all intentional wrongdoing and harm, especially from fornication with woman or man, bond or free."

Relevant portions of the oath are reproduced here. With changing times interpretation does and should change, but the crux or the nucleus of the oath should remain in revered sanctity.

Today the same oath ought probably be renamed the hypocritical oath. Can this noble profession be converted into a noble business? Earning money, but not losing one's conscience to the devil should be the guiding value. The trust fostered in the patients heart by a conscientious doctor can be the mantra to instill confidence in the public and restore the ever diminishing faith in this noble 'business'.

The nobility of a deed is judged by the intentions of the doer. Many a literary work, scripture and religious book can be quoted in this regard. We have to agree in principle that medicine was, is and shall always be considered a noble profession, at times a thankless one. Humans are very weak when they are suffering. In the hour of agony and suffering, whoever gives solace or heals becomes a 'messiah', or a supernatural power, if not God himself. Since this power has no other intention except to heal, nobility gets attached to the people who help in this type of healing. This analogy of God to mortals, in this case the doctor, makes the professional feel akin to a divine one. But there's a catch: no one is ready to take failure as the work of God - then it means that the doctor has goofed up.

Nobility has many definitions. The traits of nobility that apply to the medical profession include honourable conduct, selflessness, morally correct and chivalrous behavior, generosity and exemplary professional skills. A few more meanings could perhaps be added, but these should suffice for our purpose. Now, this is where it gets interesting. Patients, especially Indian patients, are generally very emotional, faithful and blindly loyal as far as their doctor is concerned. The iconic status of the doctor is parallel to that of a supernatural power. After a satisfactory job and when the result of the treatment is positive, a crown is invariably placed by the patients and the relatives on the doctor's head and heaps of praise are showered. This is natural of any positive outcome anywhere. The difference is when the doctor starts feeling and behaving like a supernatural power. This attitude has led to many problems and is probably the single largest cause for the change in public perceptions of the medical community that we see today.

Over the years, the outlook of the public towards doctors has changed considerably. A successful, rich doctor is not treated with great reverence for the simple reason that he is beyond the reach of a certain stratum of people. It is generally believed that he has earned his money the wrong way, by dubious means and by fleecing patients. There is a strong and deep-rooted bias in this regard in the minds of Indians. The root cause of this psyche is perhaps colonial rule and the injustice which the poor and the downtrodden experienced at the hands of their masters and employers. The same school of thought is always partial towards the weaker strata, irrespective of the negatives present in the weaker sections. The driver of a larger vehicle on the road is always the culprit despite the cyclist's blatant mistake. A rich guy is deemed to have earned his money through unscrupulous means. A swanky hospital owner has earned a lot of money because he could pump in a huge amount for upgradation by fleecing the patients. Nobody is willing to believe that the doctor has created this facility to serve the patients and may in fact have taken huge loans to do so.

The dichotomy is that it is also considered to be appropriate for a successful individual and especially a doctor to move around in a luxury car for maximum impact. When he moves around in one bought on borrowed money, he attracts allegations.

The general public is better informed now and is bolder in its allegations. Earlier the respect for a doctor never dwindled, regardless of his shortcomings. The public used to pardon the follies. Not anymore. Everybody is putting in hard labour to rise and nobody wants to be taken for a ride. It is common knowledge that the payouts made by doctors go far beyond their own practicing domains. Anybody who helps add to the consultancy practice is put on a payroll. This payout could go to people like a rickshaw driver, an ambulance driver, a bus driver or just about anyone bringing in referrals. These are the people who help set up practices for many aspiring practitioners. These are also the people who gossip and show the medical field in a poor light. A few payouts go to the fraternity and to paramedical personnel, including the local pharmacist. Anyone who gets you money faster is welcome. Age is also an important factor. A doctor is productive as long as he is in active practice. The moment he retires, there is a sharp dip in income.

This is the cruel reality.

Such competition, hard work and a problematic public interface have together combined to make the medical profession appear unattractive to many youngsters. This is why maximum earning in minimum time and securing the future first have become the mantras. With every passing year competitive exams for medical entrance are seeing a continuous fall in the number of aspirants appearing for the exam. Many of the students who graduate with an MBBS degree are venturing out towards other kinds of businesses and jobs, and not pursuing the medical profession. Does anybody counsel an individual who wants to become a first generation doctor? Apart from the competitive exams, why should a psychological analysis not be carried out? The student should be asked what his expectations from the vocation are. He should be informed of what is in store for him. If people are educated properly about these matters few would take up medicine. Instead of a flood of students it will become a trickle. If the first-ever medical graduate in the family has done well then one should go ahead.

Earlier, a medical graduate was not supposed to do anything else or to even know anything apart from his line of work. It held true for most, but the ones who ventured out and were successful still wanted to be known first as doctors. Perhaps they wanted to indicate that they were well educated and had a noble facet to their personalities. The same is not the case with an engineer graduating out of, say, IIT or a graduate of any other top school. The doctor's life is made into a comparative index. The comparison is between how he was when he started and how he is at present. The many years of hard work, the bank loans that needed to be repaid, the sleepless nights spent worrying about patients who were not doing well and the vacations cancelled because of work pressure are not taken into consideration.

The critic never takes into account the hard work behind the success, and the advanced medical treatment that is offered. The same public wants a physically fit, 24-hour alert, well-dressed, well-informed, well-read, doctor. The doctor should be at the beck and call of the patients 24 x 7 x 365 +2 days a year. He should give priority to his profession at the expense of his family and friends. He should never misbehave and should be courteous at all hours. He should be able to diagnose all ailments in every patient that he comes across and should treat every patient successfully. He should not charge much money and should be generous. He should help everybody financially. He should give credit and even be willing to forget about money owed to him by patients. He should help the patient in such ways even when the latter has rich relatives and friends. Those people are for moral support. He should forgo his fee so that the patient and relatives can spend three times the money on an event which is of social value, after the patient has recovered fully. The doctor should keep on reducing the charges whenever any prominent relative or friend surfaces. This, even if the amount has been mutually agreed on prior to the operation. The doctor should examine and treat everyone who accompanies a patient free of charge. If a doctor does not do this, he is branded a businessman. He is thought of as money-minded, etc. It is understandable that a doctor's career success may make his own professional brethren envious, but it is inexplicable when people from outside the field, who have no rivalry with him, get envious; when his patients, for instance, start harming the interests and growth of the very doctor who has treated them sincerely over the years. And yet, it is a fact that this harmonious and mutually sustaining relationship often changes overnight when the doctor's improved circumstances become evident to his patients. It is beyond comprehension why the human psyche changes so suddenly: it defies all logical reasoning and explanation. Is this why a noble profession is turning into a questionably noble business? After all, no other professional is answerable in quite same way to just about anybody. Where other professionals are concerned, their vacations are theirs, their fees and earnings are theirs, their style of doing business may be anti-national and anti-mankind, but they are not similarly held to account by all and sundry. If a less educated, less qualified individual earns more than is warranted, it is acceptable, but if the doctor is earning reasonably, it is a point of contention. If a doctor is getting decent money after decades of hard work, it is questionable, but if a less educated person from another field gets it in the first two or three years, he is considered either lucky or hard working – and rarely becomes the subject of controversy, unless there is overwhelming and obvious evidence of his having been involved in a scam of some sort! Perhaps that's why ruthlessness has set-in in the medical profession and more and more doctors are showing a callous approach to the human side of their work.

These developments are increasingly leading to relationships of mistrust, bad feelings, unfaithfulness and an increase in animosity between the healer and the patient. This scenario is more marked in larger cities, where there is survival of the fittest, and several options for treatment are available.

In balance, one must say that there are several reasons as to why the doctor-patient relationship is deteriorating by the day. It is not that either can be held solely responsible for this. No single cause, theory or answer can satisfy everybody. I believe that if inputs are gathered from people, there shall be thousands of suggestions. There will be many more explanations, defences and rebuttals of whatever is being presented. The effort here is to start a thought process and not an argument. This is only to spark off a thought process and lead to introspection. In pursuit of this, it may be worthwhile to examine another potential causative factor.

This concerns the rapid technological advancements that have characterized the field of medicine in recent years. Our metro cities began to offer world class healthcare and services. Huge investments were made to upgrade facilities. Most of the promoters were business people. The deterioration in doctor-patient relations could possibly be traced to this modernization. It is not to say that the technological advancement was unnecessary, but that it increased the disparities between the rich and the poor in terms of the kinds of treatment they could afford. The affluent did not mind paying whatever fees were asked for, especially since many among them had until then been going abroad to access advanced technologies and these now became available at a comparatively lower cost in our own country. All of this accentuated their VIP status in a very visible way. Seeing this, the venture capitalists tasted blood. Many took the trend a step further and started offering some of these high-tech medical services in smaller towns and larger non-metro cities as well. Thus the new technologies and treatment options started changing the motive for setting up hospitals – they became profit centers. Every law of doing business believes that whenever you invest money, it has to generate increased revenue – whether by volumes or margins – only then can the returns be deemed healthy. Investments made by the business class had their own calculations. For them recovery of their capital at a cost which included interest and profits was of prime concern. A target of earnings and revenue generation to be achieved in a fixed time was given to doctors. This is scary in the healthcare sector which is not a money-making proposition in the poor countries. Doctors who could ensure revenue generation at the cost of the oath and the ethics were primarily promoted. Anything one could get away with under the garb of professionalism was done. A battery of unnecessary diagnostic tests, procedures and treatment modalities were advocated. Healthcare costs thus multiplied. Doctors who based their practice on more rational medical lines were gradually eased out. From being a society of brilliant diagnosticians who adapted ingeniously to challenging infrastructural conditions and yet yielded excellent results, the country changed into a test-first and diagnose-later medical society. Whether this was justified and required is a debatable point. Medical care became world class in the developed pockets of society but affordability went down. The proportion of the population benefiting remained the same because the development and deployment of modern healthcare facilities was not balanced and well distributed – it was confined to privileged areas, metros, VIP habitats. The rate of spread into smaller towns, semi-urban and rural areas, has been very low and not so successful either. To use technology, one has to be tech-savvy, and this has been one glaring gap in the education curriculum.

The next explosion, to improve affordability, came by way of healthcare insurance. Lopsided policies with huge loopholes got implemented. Corruption at the patient, health-care provider and insurance company level soared to unimaginable heights. The companies succeeded in increasing the overhead costs of small and medium healthcare units. Externally defined mandatory minimum infrastructural criteria became essential prerequisites for insurance claims. How a reimbursement can depend primarily on the size of a hospital is a question even the best thinking minds cannot answer. If a patient has been taking treatment from a doctor at a setup which the doctor feels is adequate, who are the administrative, non-medical 'babus' to refuse reimbursement? In essence, the 'babus' are saying that the doctor does not know what is good for his patient and the patient is safe only at places where the overheads are huge and the bills are even more so. Over time, all of this led to a scenario where the bills got inflated.

The patients who had a health insurance policy, and who did not intend to go to large hospitals still paid more than what they had been paying earlier, because the benchmark of payments got higher. It is a fact that people don't generally take kindly to being co-opted into activities that help inflate others' incomes. A time came when the patients started realizing what was going on. By that time a lot of mistrust had developed. Another noteworthy factor is that the larger hospitals absorbed only the highly qualified and highly influential super-specialist moneymaker doctors and their coterie. This is a vital point in healthcare. Most of the hospitals tied up with the same set of doctors and the same set of people started representing all the hospitals – with the exception of government hospitals, which could not afford to cater to the 'page 3' of society.

A strong undercurrent of jealousy grew within the fraternity, fostered by the people who were feeling left out and ignored. A big question mark arose on the intention and nobility of the medical profession. The suspicion grew that doctors were increasingly acting selfishly and unethically. This may not be a general rule but the proportion of bad fish is increasing by the day. It is no more a case of one fish spoiling the pond. Two more factors responsible for this breach of trust are the consumer law in our country and to a certain extent the media. Consumer law is a 'cause-effect-cause' kind of a scenario. In the past, there was nothing in our country which could be used against blatant wrongdoing, negligence and the callous attitude of some doctors. Everything was taken on faith. When that faith got eroded, vengeance took over and when that happened the final nail in the coffin was driven. Inadvertently and without understanding medical nuances, the media created hype about small mishaps and so-called negligence. The media never bothered to follow up such cases and close the debate with a report on correct facts and the factual outcome of consumer courts. This acted as a catalyst. The ruthless businessman in the doctor was born. Many years of hard study and incommensurate revenues, especially in ratio to the hard work put in; no government or trust hospital support as far as the salaries are concerned; no placement in good hospitals; a lopsided demand and supply ratio in urban India: all of these combined with the understandable desire in each doctor to see himself as successful, and compelled the medical fraternity to take to dubious means. Earning in whatever way possible became the only criterion for success. Job satisfaction and conscientiousness took a back seat. A mad rush to show off wealth and power in the shape of swanky cars, exotic vacations, designer clothes and the like ensued.

This led to a casualty. Nobody in this rat race realized that the urban hospitals were attracting fewer patients now. One of the reasons for these dwindling numbers was that better centers kept on cropping up in the rural areas, and the other that the urban centers started getting saturated with more and more doctors. The supply of the doctors went up and that of patients went down because the supply of patients got distributed. This led to a panic situation. The successful ones or the hungry started creating satellite centers and started going to a multiplicity of institutions as visiting faculty. This further decreased the supply of patients and a long term recessionary impact ensued. Pressure to maintain expensive lifestyles prompted more irregularities leading to the present situation. This peculiarity got a bit exaggerated because of the migration of population and inhabitation along caste lines. There are areas where specific doctors rule the roost owing to the fact they belong to a certain caste or social community group. Proficiency in the profession is in no way related to the success they enjoy. The cause-effect-cause theory got ratified and doctor-patient relations took a further battering. Thus the noble profession yielded to noble business. The noble business too is getting eroded resulting in a fight to survive, which means survival of the fittest.

Any overt or covert act now is directly or indirectly related to earning, so a cut-throat business wears the mask of a noble profession and anything is pardonable.

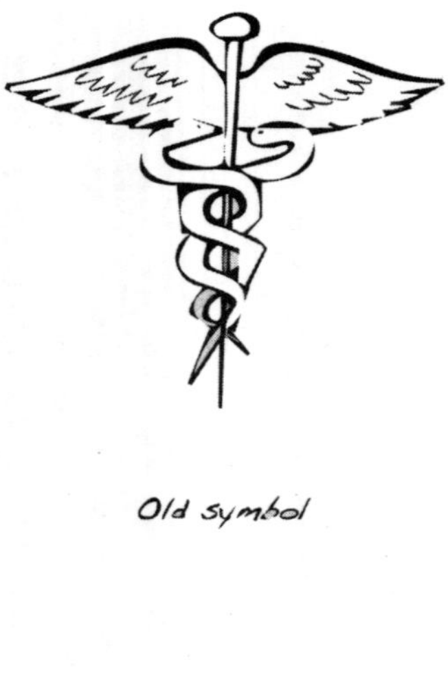

Old symbol

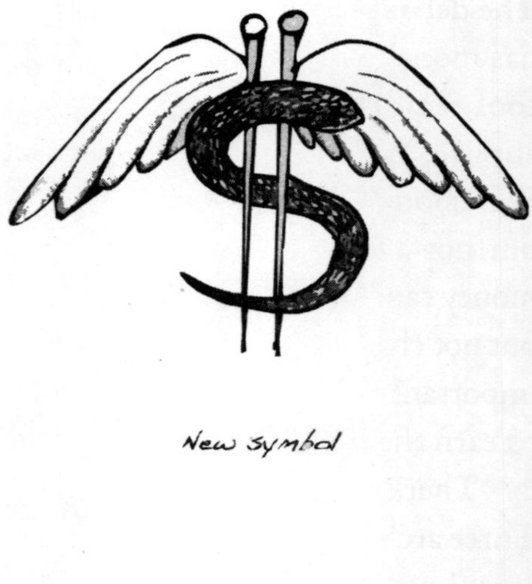

New symbol

MONEY IS MERIT

The definition of a successful person in today's world is 'one who has money and knows how to flaunt it'. Money is a very powerful tool required to survive in a society where only the fittest can survive. With money a person can buy anything, or so he thinks. Somebody wrote in beautiful verses that money can buy a house, but not a home: money can buy amusement but not happiness; money can buy medicine but not health and money can buy etiquette but not character. Most of us know this; still we attach the maximum importance to money and respect a moneyed man. How he has come to earn the money is no more a consideration. This is a sad truth.

There are numerous ways of earning money and getting rich. Three archetypal methods are: the way of the rabbit, the way of the tortoise and the way of the fox. The individual characteristics of each animal are well known. These animal characteristics are symbolically applicable in the real life scenario of a medical professional. It's the foxy way of becoming rich which is leading to the decadence of the profession.

The tortoise in the fable won at a slow and steady pace. Similarly, in earlier times, life was led at a comfortable pace. But in today's world, any game which entails hard work, takes a long time and has an uncertain outcome has very few takers. One might also take the analogy of the most popular game in our country – cricket. Test matches were very popular in the olden days. The idea was to savour the fine points of the game and equally to enjoy the weather, the picnic-like atmosphere and the evening parties. In much the same way money used to be earned at a slow but steady pace. Even the opportunity to spend or to multiply the money was limited. The rich professionals did not know where to plough the money back for quick returns, nor, perhaps, did they think of these quite as much.

Over time, the preference shifted to faster and shorter games. A 50-over game in cricket became more popular and very recently 20-20 game is catching up. Tests became boring and quick-fire competitions became the order of the day. Similarly, in business, the zeal to make quick money grew. Money earned fast, in huge proportions became the mantra. Money multiplication avenues increased. Earnings could be ploughed back into other fields which offered multiplication of money at a faster rate. A target of retirement was set based on that fast earning. Life's pleasurable experiences were ignored or neglected to realize the targets. This is the rabbit way of earning, fast but not dubious. It is devoid of the pleasures that life gives and fraught with dangers, though the thrill is there. This is the current scenario in most of the professions.

The one way of earning which is regrettable is the way of the fox. The fox is known for its speed, cunning and shrewdness. Doctors who make money this way are unprofessional. There are no scruples involved and no regret or remorse. Initially a few professionals joined this category, but with time, their numbers multiplied rapidly. Good deeds in life take a long time to bring fame and it takes one bad deed to lose everything. At times, it may just take a few seconds to lose everything. One false move and years of hard work goes down the drain. Yet more and more people risk this negative outcome rather than letting honesty prevail. This means that the bad deeds get recognition faster and on a larger platform. The minority of wrongdoers get the undeserved attention faster. The general public then starts painting everyone with the same brush. This has been going on for many years. What started many years back has now become a phenomenon with the majority pointing fingers at the doctors. This has made the relationship go sour.

Half-baked knowledge presented in the magazines, newspapers and other modes of communication, is converting every Tom, Dick and Harry into a medically savvy, well-informed individual. Modern means of communication have shrunk the world and everything in the medical world is available at the touch of a button. A doctor's years of experience and the application of that experience while making decisions regarding treatment have become devalued. Whether this is correct or not is debatable. Certain legal acts have added fuel to the fire.

A centuries-old relationship of mutual trust has deteriorated drastically. Yet neither the sufferer nor the healer seems able to undo the damage. There are shortcomings with both and these need to be addressed. The moot point is: who bells the cat? The problem may diminish if the human angle in treatment is reintroduced. But this apart, introspection by the medical fraternity and identification of the factors which have led to this mistrust are very important. The quick foxes have to be exposed. Who these quick foxes are is something that is largely known to the medical fraternity, but there has been a tendency in the profession to close ranks and, in effect, shield such persons.

An effective system of checks and balances has to be evolved to see that patients are not exploited for the purpose of earning more money. If a reasonable option is available, the patient should be told about it. In other words, the Right to Information Act should be applied intelligently as a tool for ensuring this. Quite obviously, I am not suggesting anything that would compromise on the quality of treatment, and I am sure the medical fraternity would understand this. What is being advocated here is that the choice of treatment should be governed by a scientific rationale and not by monetary considerations. There should not be one set of standards for close relatives and friends and another set for the paying public. A very interesting but deplorable and nauseating episode comes to mind. This dates back to the time when I was the treasurer of a Medical Association. When my two-year tenure was coming to an end, we ran a questionnaire. It was in two parts. A case study was presented and ninety-nine percent of the doctors responding recommended an operation as the desirable form of treatment. When the second part of the questionnaire was circulated which asked what the treatment modality should be if the patient was your own father, ninety-nine percent of the doctors replied that a conservative trial was advisable before contemplating surgery.

The quick foxes may be an outcome of the system which is slowly being taken over by money-minded, non-medical businessmen and administrators. The rich businessman and entrepreneur creates the best working places and employs good professionals. As the doctor gets trapped in working at the best places where the elite of society come, he is forced to adopt the tricks of the trade. The quick money game is run in the name of these credulous doctors. These naïve brethren of the fraternity end up being puppets in somebody else's hands. Professionally competent people who know nothing beyond patient welfare get exploited. Revenue earners are invited to patronize hospitals. A different set of rules and sweeping powers are offered to them. Targets are given to these main doctors who become the power lobbies and earners of the hospital. Little does this gullible set of doctors realize that it is their reputation which is at stake. Mind you, it is not as if they get the lion's share of the profits either. To take an example, in a bill of forty-five thousand for a patient operated on for piles, the doctor gets only twelve thousand rupees, and this money is received only after 45 days. There is a pattern of deduction which is variable for different doctors. Nobody is answerable if there is a discrepancy. If a rebate or waiver is to be given to the patient during the final settlement of the patient's huge bill, the deductions are made from the doctor's professional fees and rarely from the hospital's bills. There are no fixed formulas for deduction. A few administrators may refute this charge but the reality can be proven. Still the brethren who yield to these powerful money lobbies do not realize their folly. The administrators patronize and promote the ones who toe their line. No doubt a good earning potential is realized and a hand in glove policy gets initiated.

I was working in one of the premier institutes of Gujarat where I was made a superintendent without my consent. I left my job within three months of that appointment and started looking for other avenues. During that tenure I learned a lot of things which are not to be found in any medical text. Even a course in MBA at a premier institute cannot teach those things. An episode which happened many years back is so fresh in my mind that even after twenty years I feel as if it happened yesterday.

A target was given to a group of competent doctors, all young and dynamic. A patient with secondaries (cancer spread) in the liver diagnosed without any room for doubt by the radiologist was subjected to another eight thousand rupees worth of tests to provide the same diagnosis. The patient was first subjected to a blind needle biopsy. The diagnosis given by the pathologist was inconclusive. The patient was charged for the procedure. He was then subjected to a sonography-guided tissue biopsy. 'Secondaries from an adenocarcinoma, (a variety of stomach cancer)' was the pathologist report. The patient was charged again. A C.T. scan was advised to look for the primary growth. Diagnosis: secondaries in the liver; primary cancer growth in the stomach. The patient was then advised open biopsy from the primary site, to assess operability and to decide the course of treatment in stage four cancers. A stage four cancer has very limited options and convincing the patient of anything contrary to this is dubious. The patient was given an estimate of another ten thousand after he had paid rupees eight thousand at different places. The patient changed the hospital. He went with the advice of the doctor who told him that nothing much could be done. Before leaving, the patient complained of the loss of trust he had for all the doctors in the hospital. Little did he realize that the doctors were like bonded labour. Let the fraternity decide whether this was done for professional reasons or just for money. I must highlight another episode. A rich and famous person woke up in the middle of the night complaining of chest pain. One of the best physicians, a blue eyed boy of the management who was ever willing to oblige at odd hours without even charging appropriate fees, was summoned to his bungalow. The patient's blood pressure and electrocardiogram turned out to be normal. He was given anti-acidity medicines with a sleeping pill. He slept well. However, in cardiology, protocols of chest pain investigation are such that any pain in the chest is considered to be heart related, until proved otherwise. The patient visited the hospital as per the advice. The repeat cardiogram was normal. Blood enzyme studies sent to the lab turned out to be normal. He was nonetheless asked to get echocardiography done. It turned out to be normal. A final test called stress test or TMT was requested by the doctors and the patient complied. This too was absolutely normal. A heart ailment was ruled out as a possible cause of the pain. Nonetheless, angiography was advised. In those days angiography could itself lead to complications. It is after all an invasive procedure. Unfortunately the patient succumbed during that test, to the shock and dismay of every treating and non-treating doctor who was following the case or hearing about it. Needless to say, the case became a cautionary tale in the folklore of medical enthusiasm. It became a point of teasing between the fresh, dynamic protagonists of overzealous treatments and the older conservative antagonists of these new modalities. A text book of surgery says that a "living problem is better than a death certificate." In this case, the patient didn't even have a problem. An overenthusiastic and overzealous approach led to this unfortunate end. In the olden days angiography had a definite, but a very low mortality rate. The decision of guilty or not guilty is perennially debatable.

There are several such examples where the dividing line is difficult to draw, between valid investigations and unnecessary investigations with a commercial motive. To what extent does an action by a doctor in the course of treating a patient qualify under the fox category? A few other examples cited here can throw some light on the issue.

A patient has excruciating pain in the region of the kidney and ureters. She experiences pain while passing urine and has nausea as well. An ultrasound shows a four to five mm stone pouting out of the ureteral orifice (opening). It is very evident that the stone is going to pop out at any minute and the issue that needs to be tackled is the patient's pain. A simple pain killer injection can take care of the issue. A somewhat more commercial but still relatively benevolent piece of advice is to infuse intravenous fluids and a diuretic. The fact is, a forceful push given by the pressure of urine normally expels the stone, but the infusion certainly helps. But the advice given on the basis of unscrupulous monetary considerations is an immediate operation without a delay of even one hour. A delay will expel the stone and the patient may ask for postponement of the operation because the pain subsides. That is why it is touted as a dire emergency. The patient is in extreme pain and is no position to decline any advice given by the doctor. Whether it is right or wrong to advise an operation is at the very least a subject for debate. This is where foresight and experience come in. It is not when to operate, but when not to operate that should be the guiding principle.

Fever is the single most challenging clinical entity. The public wants a fast cure and the best doctor is considered to be the one who provides relief from it the fastest way. Medicines which work on all fevers whether infective, viral, malarial or protozoal are started simultaneously. No thought is given to whether these are indicated or are potentially harmful and preferably avoidable, or to the fact that unnecessary use of certain medicines could lead to resistance, thereby reducing their effectiveness when they are actually needed. Laurels are showered on the doctor who magically cures the fever. Unfortunately medicine is not about magic. Miracles perhaps, but not magic. Miracles are conceivable because after all, nature is the ultimate healer and nature is often miraculous.

The sad part is that many doctors are well aware that all this is happening. The realization has to dawn in the minds of doctors that this approach is boomeranging on the entire medical fraternity. An ignorant attitude, and a callous attitude of 'I couldn't care less because I am not a part of it' is damaging the minds and reputations of even the honest doctors. Several such examples get circulated as gossip when people sit and share their experiences and all doctors are judged according to the standards set by their less worthy peers.

An NRI lady visited her doctor who had operated on her a year earlier, to check whether everything was fine. The doctor who had conducted the surgery was not available. The lady went to somebody who had a hospital in the neighbourhood. This doctor after examining her said that she had a fibroid in her uterus. Being familiar with technology trends, the doctor also added that the latest method to treat such cases was laser technology. The NRI went out amazed and rather bewildered. She had been operated on a year earlier for the fibroid in her uterus and her uterus had already been removed in the process! When she went back to the original doctor after getting her sonography done, it was absolutely normal and no further intervention was required. What will happen to the opinion of this NRI regarding Indian doctors? Won't she share her experience with others? Wouldn't this incident mean that similar stories of wrongdoing by other doctors would gain in credibility, regardless of their veracity? These incidents must warn us that the actions of one unethical doctor affect all; the whole group loses professional credibility. We can no longer afford to ignore the wrong practices of other doctors; we must demand a code of conduct and adherence to it.

Other unethical practices relate to exhibiting success. Blatantly unethical medical advertising is in particular an area that deserves greater scrutiny. Such advertising takes many forms, direct and indirect. One way of signifying success is by attending conferences as faculty, chairperson, moderator or speaker. In all of these, no opportunity is lost in projecting the 'I' factor. A second but less effective way is to trumpet one's achievements in scientific journals and medical association bulletins. This is often resorted to when any new technology is obtained. Successful doctors in our country have also used other ingenious methods. One such gentleman ensured that heaps of footwear were always lying outside his clinic premises, day in and day out, throughout the year. This was to make onlookers believe that there was always a rush of patients. Our friend also ensured that several cars and two wheelers were parked outside the hospital. Naturally there was a tie-up with a garage. The rotation of vehicles was a must for authenticity. The message sought to be conveyed was that work never ended in the hospital, that there was an endless stream of patients. Outpatient appointments were given in such a way that one or other goodwill ambassador or sycophant was always amongst the people waiting outside. These people had a role to play and they did it voluntarily. They sang the doctor's praises loudly and frequently before the assembled audience of other patients.

Another doctor routinely sent patients who were to be operated on to visit, on one pretext or another, other patients he had operated on successfully. Alternatively, he ensured that the patient to be operated on ended up talking to another patient who had not got the desired or promised result from an arch rival of the doctor's. Whether this is business strategy or fox-like earning is once again open to debate. God only knows what will happen if the trend follows cricket even further and becomes the medical equivalent of a 20/20 match! Nowadays even 50-over matches are becoming obsolete.

While debating issues of this kind, it is pertinent to think about the causative factors. It would be unfair to fix responsibility only on the doctors for this. Which human being is above the desire for luxury? Which mortal does not succumb to easy virtues and shortcuts to making money? Whether such factors should or should not affect people is not the issue here. The point is: who is responsible for bringing about this change in a naïve professional? Is it the patient? Is it the pharmaceutical industry, which patronizes only the successful, and shows them a life of easy luxury? Yes, to a certain extent everybody is partially responsible – in fact we all have collective responsibility for what has come to pass. However, the individual who matters the most is the doctor himself. His proportion in the responsibility is the highest. After window shopping for treatment avenues, patients settle on a particular doctor. A price is fixed after haggling and the best rates are offered. The patient and the relatives want the doctor to do his best and not compromise on anything. The best disposable items are requested to be used. Everything goes according to a perfect plan. Nearer the time to pay, a tremendous amount of pressure is brought to bear on the doctor from different quarters and a discount or rebate is sought. If it is not given the patient indirectly hints at withdrawal of patronage. Isn't the doctor supposed to devise ways to overcome this nonsense? The same patient after getting a rebate goes around boasting in his social circles about the huge amount he spent on a certain treatment. For him it is a matter of pride; for the doctor who has undercharged it is a matter of disgust. Shouldn't the doctor tackle this disgusting menace? A few patients add their eating and entertaining expenditure to make up the total cost of treatment. This is a cost which is totally avoidable but in our country patients tend to be visited by large numbers of friends and relatives expecting hospitality. They expect to be taken care of. These overheads are an important reason for patients bargaining with doctors to reduce the actual medical component of their treatment related expenditure. Besides, after getting a rebate from the hapless doctor the financially challenged patient also has, on successfully leaving the hospital, to blow a huge amount on 'post-medical' social obligations. No friend or relative comes forward to help him in either scenario. All they do is to pressurize the doctor to reduce his billing. Even the rich relatives run away when billing is in process. Therefore the doctor does what he has to do!

In the olden days kings used to decide who was to be paid what. Experience, skill and the level of difficulty of the job were not necessarily the criteria for determining payment. This monarchical tendency continues in the medical profession. The insurance companies have taken the role of erstwhile monarchs. The rates a doctor should charge are now being dictated by these companies. When an individual applies for a housing loan, does the bank decide how much the carpenter or the mason will get? A company which knows little about medicine appoints a medical graduate to lay down policies regarding treatment and billing. When the bills are presented, lame excuses and flimsy grounds are created to delay the remuneration or reject the amount asked. It is ironic but true. A doctor sitting on an insurance company's chair should be helping doctors, especially since he knows fully well what happens in a lot of operations, and yet he generally behaves in exactly the opposite manner under instructions from his employers! An example of this silly thought process can be gauged from the fact that the cost fixed for a uterus removal operation where the size is normal to marginally enlarged is the same as that for a uterus removal where there are multiple tumors (fibroids), simply because the medical name for both the operations is hysterectomy. Technically the first of these procedures can be completed, by an experienced doctor, in around forty five minutes while the other would take the same doctor as much as ninety minutes. Is this then not unfair to the doctors? A mason gets paid by the type of work and number of hours he spends on the job, so does a consultant of any other branch. We are skilled, and we devote time, but we have a different set of rules crafted by society at large.

To try to enroll in an insurance company has become an exercise in futility if one follows the correct path. The criteria to get onto the network of hospitals for cashless benefits for the patient are set by the company. The company is more worried about the well being of the patient than the doctor! The four main general insurance companies have appointed multiple third party administrators who have a minimal presence in most of the states except where the head office is located. There are no criteria for the company office. It's only the financial clout of the promoter that counts. Once appointed, the third party administrators or TPAs start flexing their muscles. It is natural that for them it is a business proposition. They have a regulatory body above them which is uniform. But while enrolling the doctors they make the doctor pledge that he will give a discount to their patients. It is like taking a cut. Whether this discount goes to the patient should be the subject of a probe. To get the bill passed within the stipulated time is a monumental task. It is not my intention to cast aspersions on the integrity of the managers but rumours are rife about rampant corruption in such cases. Getting enlisted on a scheme in which cashless benefits are passed on to the patients takes a lot of effort of the other kind. Since the patient believes that cashless hospitalization is a hassle-free option, the motivation amongst doctors for getting on the board of TPA network hospitals is high. Only the network enlisted hospitals of the TPA get the facility of cashless treatment. There are approximately 45 to 50 TPAs already and being on all of them is good business for the doctors. A lesser known fact is that to get on the network hospital or to get the bill passed after being on the network or otherwise, a lot of palms may have to be greased. Is the doctor supposed to do this, especially to enroll or take his rightfully earned money? In spite of the apex court's ruling that a maximum of 90 days should be the time to settle accounts, compliance with the order is negligible. The reason for inflated bills is that a lot of payouts as well as delays in getting payments have irked the medical fraternity. Whoever conceived the TPA route offloaded his headache onto someone else. It did not help in achieving anything but led to the creation of more jobs. Agents and touts who collude with the insurance personnel have mushroomed. A lot of jobs have sprung up in hospitals to take care of insurance related hassles. Great for the job market but a total fiasco for the medical industry.

Corruption in the medical industry crept in most imperceptibly – I cannot say it was never there, but it is certainly very deplorable and disgusting and should be stopped. Are the doctors responsible for these policies? They are the victims who have devised ways to overcome unwanted obstacles. The 'inspector raj' has slowly invaded the noble field of medicine because of the lopsided government policies and social practices. These days doctors have to deal with a huge number of such inspectors: pollution control inspectors, agencies monitoring female foeticide, labour inspectors, provident fund inspectors, service tax inspectors, income tax inspectors, consumer court inspectors and police inspectors. Of course, the medical field is undergoing a change like any other industry but it should not be at the cost of the patient or the doctor. Nobody realizes that things were very easy in the olden days and that's why the attitude of the doctor was milder. We hope that things do not get worse from here on but if they do, the responsibility for this must be placed firmly on the shoulders of a wide range of stakeholders.

MEDICAL CAREER STILL SURVIVES

Any vocation even remotely connected with science in our country has always been a coveted profession, including medicine and engineering, which enjoy top positions in the professional hierarchy. In my days medicine and engineering were the two professions that every parent wanted his child to pursue. My parents never pressurized me or my younger brother about our studies. We were given the best of education in the best of schools but were far from being pampered children. Even at that early age I had my dreams, but becoming a doctor was not one of them. My father was a strict disciplinarian. He was particular about two things, correct attire and etiquette. Owing to this kind of austere background I always wanted to be in a glamorous job and was inclined towards hotel management. I thought I was good at managing the parties and functions that used to take place as I was growing up.

Before the time came for me to have to choose an educational stream in the 11th class, we shifted to Washington at the end of the seventies. I joined the local school there and started pursuing my high school from the 9th grade. Though a rather mediocre student in India, I started excelling in that school in the U.S. When I attained the legal age to work in the state of Virginia, of 15 years and 8 months, I decided to take up a job. The jobs that were available and suited the school timings were those of a newspaper delivery boy, or odd jobs in restaurants and gas stations. I had to deliver 'The Washington Post' in the early hours and I hated the job, but I plodded on because my father allowed me to do only this job. However he later agreed to let me do any other job I wished, and soon I was working in a restaurant. I worked hard as a dishwasher, bartender, utility man and waiter and then changed jobs and worked in a sandwich franchise which has outlets all over the world today. I also worked at a gas station (or petrol pump, as we call them in India). The main task was pumping gas but in the spare time when there were no customers, the gas station roads were to be built and maintenance work such as wall painting was required to be done. This I did while excelling in my studies and getting a GPA of 3.8. As I was nearing graduation, and looking at hotel management as my area of specialization, my father said that he wanted me to go back to India and study medicine. I submitted to his wishes because he insisted on this and couldn't relate to my hotel management fantasy. Not that getting into a medical college was a cake walk, but I succeeded and became a doctor. I completed an M.S. in surgery, and later on did an advanced diploma course in hospital administration. In between I underwent urology training for three years at a premier institute of Ahmedabad under the tutorship of one of the most revered urologists of that era. Now I have a successful practice. I practice in the field of gastrointestinal surgery and have an expertise in urological diseases also. The dreams were always there. Since I was the first doctor in the family from my mother's side, my parents took a lot of pride in my profession perhaps more than I did myself. Being a first generation doctor and no one to guide you is a difficult business. I married my college girlfriend, who is an 'ardhangini' in every sense of the word. She is an M.D. in gynaecology. As long as we were both under the umbrella of our bosses and teachers, we felt that the profession we had chosen was the best and were confident of making our dreams come true. Then it came time to say goodbye to the alma mater and move on. Being bonded candidates we took up jobs in a rural hospital very near Ahmedabad and spent two years there. There was both job satisfaction and a reasonable amount of money. Then we moved on to Ahmedabad and set up a rudimentary kind of hospital in 1991. That was all our means would permit. We thought that hard work was the formula to success. I took up a job to supplement our meager income. We had to rely on bank loans and pay the exorbitant interest prevalent at that time. It was an achievement for us especially because we had decided to go it all the way on our own and not trouble our parents at all. The first instalment gave us a shock. Our earnings in the preceding three months had been Rs 18000 and the first instalment came to Rs 36,000. It wiped out all our savings and a little bit of my wife's jewellery. The first paying patient who delivered a child at our place was in December of 1991. It was tough, treading the ethical path. Practising in an unknown area, having no referral support from surrounding doctors and no financial support took its toll on our patience. There were times we thought of closing down the hospital and moving on. We even tried the parochial route; since this was Gujarat, I asked my wife to practice in her maiden Gujarati name, thinking it would attract more patients on the basis of regional affiliations. We tried all sorts of things to keep ourselves afloat, but nonetheless, patient footfalls were few and far between. We firmly believed though, that a doctor's path is difficult at the start and that these hardships would slowly get over. If we were good in what we did and how we did it, then success was bound to happen. It took seven years of struggle to get reasonable results. From 1998, my wife came into the reckoning as a good doctor and patients from all economic strata started coming to her at our hospital. Then came a phase when consultations were happening but they did not convert themselves into surgeries. Even the friends who believed in our capabilities would not get operated on or admitted. The setup we had was such that patients would not go in for major surgeries. Because of that we renovated the premises three times and even expanded it a year ago. Now 'Samarpan Hospital' has a modern look. The immense amount of problems that we faced during the expansion is a long story in itself. In fact I began writing this book because of the problems we faced. We were good doctors, but not marketing experts. Because of our modest startup status in the profession we had no locus standi to question any wrongdoing. The series of renovations and expansions have been very educative experiences on how to get work done and all that happens in our industry. Having seen and heard the different things happening around me and having escaped the easy option of falling prey to that kind of practice, I thought of writing this book on doctors. A minority of my unthinking fraternity is responsible for the downhill trend that seems evident in this noble profession. A few lines by Sir Zachary Cope and some others by Sir Robert Grove Hutchison that are quoted in our textbook of surgery should be highlighted here:

"A disease is sometimes diagnosed,
But oft the best attempts will meet with sad and sorrowful defeat,
So let us take good advice, examine once, examine twice,
Examine from the head to toe, before you dare to diagnose,
More harm is done because we do not look; above all do not spot,

Because we think we know a lot,
Spot diagnosis you should hate, until we are a doctor great,
By then, of course, we will have some lessons that we daren't"

These lines have a profound meaning for all clinicians. On a similar note, Sir Hutchison says:

"From inability to let well alone; from too much zeal for the new and contempt for what is old; from putting knowledge before wisdom, science before art, and cleverness before common sense, from treating patients as cases, and from making the cure of the disease more grievous than the endurance of the same, Good Lord, deliver us."

These quotes are old and the younger generation with its new ways of thinking may not agree with them. Science has progressed by leaps and bounds. A paradigm shift has happened. It is "I treat and I cure" now. However the irony is that a cure for diseases like the common cold has still not been found. Science has fantastic treatments for all the symptoms, but the disease has not been eradicated. There are many such diseases and new ones are emerging as well. Better treatment modalities and improvement in critical care is significant, but the disease stays.

As in the world of fashion, everything gets repeated after a few years. There are even some treatment modalities these days that represent a revival of the older ways of treatment. Therefore old is still gold and the deep meaning holds true for any generation.

I have tried in this little book to look at the seamy side of the medical profession in a lighter vein with malice towards none. I count myself as a part of the entire system. I blame the system and not the individual who falls prey to it. All I want to do now is to wake up and work together with my medical brethren, unite for a clean and ethical medical fraternity.

CODE OF MEDICAL ETHICS

The prime reason for putting this chapter at the end of the book is to highlight the fact that the book contains no chapter which is beyond the realm of the code of ethics. The code of ethics is a government notification. The relevant parts of the code are recreated here. This may reignite the thought process in the few who have lost the path of honesty. This may serve as a catalyst to the few who followed it but are prone to change for more materialistic gains and to the rest it may serve as knowledge. A lot of us do not know what this code of ethics says. This is what the gazette says:

The prime object of the medical profession is to render service to humanity; reward or financial gain is a subordinate concession. Whosoever chooses this profession, assumes the obligation to conduct himself in accordance with its ideals. A physician should be an upright man, instructed in the art of healings. He shall keep himself pure in character and be diligent in caring for the sick; he should be modest, sober, patient, prompt in discharging his duty without anxiety; conducting himself with propriety in his profession and in all the actions of his life.

No person other than a doctor having qualification recognized by Medical Council of India and registered with Medical Council of India/State Medical Council(s) is allowed to practice Modern system of Medicine or Surgery. A person obtaining qualification in any other system of Medicine is not allowed to practice Modern system of Medicine in any form.

The Principal objective of the medical profession is to render service to humanity with full respect for the dignity of profession and man. Physicians should merit the confidence of patients entrusted to their care, rendering to each a full measure of service and devotion. Physicians should try continuously to improve medical knowledge and skills and should make available to their patients and colleagues the benefits of their professional attainments. The physician should practice methods of healing founded on scientific basis and should not associate professionally with anyone who violates this principle. The honoured ideals of the medical profession imply that the responsibilities of the physician extend not only to individuals but also to society.

A Physician should expose, without fear or favour, incompetent or corrupt, dishonest or unethical conduct on the part of members of the profession.

The physician, engaged in the practice of medicine shall give priority to the interests of patients. The personal financial interests of a physician should not conflict with the medical interests of patients. A physician should announce his fees before rendering service and not after the operation or treatment is under way. Remuneration received for such services should be in the form and amount specifically announced to the patient at the time the service is rendered. It is unethical to enter into a contract of "no cure no payment". Physician rendering service on behalf of the state shall refrain from anticipating or accepting any consideration.

Though a physician is not bound to treat each and every person asking his services, he should not only be ever ready to respond to the calls of the sick and the injured, but should be mindful of the high character of his mission and the responsibility he discharges in the course of his professional duties. In his treatment, he should never forget that the health and the lives of those entrusted to his care depend on his skill and attention. A physician should endeavour to add to the comfort of the sick by making his visits at the hour indicated to the patients. A physician advising a patient to seek service of another physician is acceptable, however, in case of emergency a physician must treat the patient. No physician shall arbitrarily refuse treatment to a patient. However for good reason, when a patient is suffering from an ailment which is not within the range of experience of the treating physician, the physician may refuse treatment and refer the patient to another physician.

Medical practitioner having any incapacity detrimental to the patient or which can affect his performance vis-à-vis the patient is not permitted to practice his profession.

The physician should neither exaggerate nor minimize the gravity of a patient's condition. He should ensure himself that the patient, his relatives or his responsible friends have such knowledge of the patient's condition as will serve the best interests of the patient and the family.

A physician is free to choose whom he will serve. He should, however, respond to any request for his assistance in an emergency. Once having undertaken a case, the physician should not neglect the patient, nor should he withdraw from the case without giving adequate notice to the patient and his family. Provisionally or fully registered medical practitioner shall not willfully commit an act of negligence that may deprive his patient or patients from necessary medical care.

However in case of serious illness and in doubtful or difficult conditions, the physician should request consultation, but under any circumstances such consultation should be justifiable and in the interest of the patient only and not for any other consideration.

Consulting pathologists / radiologists or asking for any other diagnostic Lab investigation should be done judiciously and not in a routine manner.

In every consultation, the benefit to the patient is of foremost importance. All physicians engaged in the case should be frank with the patient and his attendants.

Utmost punctuality should be observed by a physician in making themselves available for consultations.

All statements to the patient or his representatives should take place in the presence of the consulting physicians, except as otherwise agreed. The disclosure of the opinion to the patient or his relatives or friends shall rest with the medical attendant.

Differences of opinion should not be divulged unnecessarily but when there is irreconcilable difference of opinion the circumstances should be frankly and impartially explained to the patient or his relatives or friends. It would be opened to them to seek further advice as they so desire.

No decision should restrain the attending physician from making such subsequent variations in the treatment if any unexpected change occurs, but at the next consultation, reasons for the variations should be discussed / explained. The same privilege, with its obligations, belongs to the consultant when sent for in an emergency during the absence of attending physician. The attending physician may prescribe medicine at any time for the patient, whereas the consultant may prescribe only in case of emergency or as an expert when called for.

When a patient is referred to a specialist by the attending physician, a case summary of the patient should be given to the specialist, who should communicate his opinion in writing to the attending physician.

A physician shall clearly display his fees and other charges on the board of his chamber and/or the hospitals he is visiting. Prescription should also make clear if the Physician himself dispensed any medicine.

A physician shall write his name and designation in full along with registration particulars in his prescription letter head.

Note: In Government hospital where the patient-load is heavy, the name of the prescribing doctor must be written below his/her signature.

Whenever a physician requests another physician to attend his patients during his temporary absence from his practice, professional courtesy requires the acceptance of such appointment only when he has the capacity to discharge the additional responsibility along with his / her other duties. The physician acting under such an appointment should give the utmost consideration to the interests and reputation of the absent physician and all such patients should be restored to the care of the latter upon his/her return.

When it becomes the duty of a physician occupying an official position to see and report upon an illness or injury, he should communicate to the physician in attendance so as to give him an option of being present. The medical officer / physician occupying an official position should avoid remarks upon the diagnosis or the treatment that has been adopted.

Soliciting of patients directly or indirectly, by a physician, by a group of physicians or by institutions or organisations is unethical. A physician shall not make use of him / her (or his / her name) as subject of any form or manner of advertising or publicity through any mode either alone or in conjunction with others which is of such a character as to invite attention to him or to his professional position, skill, qualification, achievements, attainments, specialities, appointments, associations, affiliations or honours and/or of such character as would ordinarily result in his self aggrandisement. A physician shall not give to any person, whether for compensation or otherwise, any approval, recommendation, endorsement, certificate, report or statement with respect of any drug, medicine, nostrum remedy, surgical, or therapeutic article, apparatus or appliance or any commercial product or article with respect of any property, quality or use thereof or any test, demonstration or trial thereof, for use in connection with his name, signature, or photograph in any form or manner of advertising through any mode nor shall he boast of cases, operations, cures or remedies or permit the publication of report thereof through any mode. A medical practitioner is however permitted to make a formal announcement in press regarding the following:

(1) On starting practice.
(2) On change of type of practice.
(3) On changing address.
(4) On temporary absence from duty.
(5) On resumption of another practice.
(6) On succeeding to another practice.
(7) Public declaration of charges.

Printing of self photograph, or any such material of publicity in the letter head or on sign board of the consulting room or any such clinical establishment shall be regarded as acts of self advertisement and unethical conduct on the part of the physician. However, printing of sketches, diagrams, picture of human system shall not be treated as unethical.

A physician may patent surgical instruments, appliances and medicine or Copyright applications, methods and procedures. However, it shall be unethical if the benefits of such patents or copyrights are not made available in situations where the interest of large population is involved.

A physician should not run an open shop for sale of medicine for dispensing prescriptions prescribed by doctors other than himself or for sale of medical or surgical appliances. It is not unethical for a physician to prescribe or supply drugs, remedies or appliances as long as there is no exploitation of the patient. Drugs prescribed by a physician or brought from the market for a patient should explicitly state the proprietary formulae as well as generic name of the drug.

A physician shall not give, solicit, or receive nor shall he offer to give solicit or receive, any gift, gratuity, commission or bonus in consideration of or return for the referring, recommending or procuring of any patient for medical, surgical or other treatment. A physician shall not directly or indirectly, participate in or be a party to act of division, transference, assignment, subordination, rebating, splitting or refunding of any fee for medical, surgical or other treatment.

Provisions of the above paragraph shall apply with equal force to the referring, recommending or procuring by a physician or any person, specimen or material for diagnostic purposes or other study / work. Nothing in this section, however, shall prohibit payment of salaries by a qualified physician to other duly qualified person rendering medical care under his supervision.

The prescribing or dispensing by a physician of secret remedial agents of which he does not know the composition, or the manufacture or promotion of their use is unethical and as such prohibited. All the drugs prescribed by a physician should always carry a proprietary formula and clear name.

Practicing euthanasia shall constitute unethical conduct. However on specific occasion, the question of withdrawing supporting devices to sustain cardio-pulmonary function even after brain death, shall be decided only by a team of doctors and not merely by the treating physician alone. A team of doctors shall declare withdrawal of support system. Such team shall consist of the doctor in charge of the patient, Chief Medical Officer / Medical Officer in charge of the hospital and a doctor nominated by the in-charge of the hospital from the hospital staff or in accordance with the provisions of the Transplantation of Human Organ Act, 1994.

The registered medical practitioner shall not refuse on religious grounds alone to give assistance in or conduct of sterility, birth control, circumcision and medical termination of Pregnancy when there is medical indication, unless the medical practitioner feels himself/herself incompetent to do so.

Before performing an operation, the physician should obtain in writing the consent from the husband or wife, parent or guardian in the case of minor, or the patient himself as the case may be. In an operation which may result in sterility the consent of both husband and wife is needed.

A Physician shall not use touts or agents for procuring patients.

A Physician shall not claim to be specialist unless he has a special qualification in that branch.

www.goodtimesbooks.com

Have you enjoyed the book?

We hope this book has helped you in

Rediscovering The New World

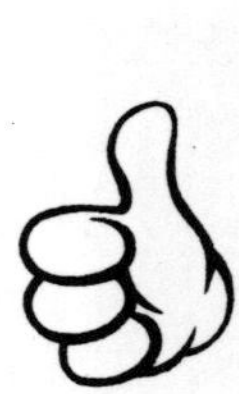